Non-prescription Medicines

Third edition

Alan Nathan

BPharm, BA, FRPharmS

Freelance pharmacy writer and consultant
London, UK

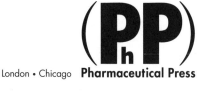

London • Chicago   **Pharmaceutical Press**

Published by the Pharmaceutical Press
An imprint of RPS Publishing

1 Lambeth High Street, London SE1 7JN, UK
100 South Atkinson Road, Suite 206, Grayslake, Il 60030-7820, USA

© Pharmaceutical Press 2006

 is a trade mark of RPS Publishing

RPS Publishing is the publishing organisation of the
Royal Pharmaceutical Society of Great Britain

First edition 1998
Second edition 2002
Reprinted 2005
Third edition 2006

Typeset by Type Study, Scarborough, North Yorkshire
Printed in Great Britain by TJ International, Padstow, Cornwall

ISBN-10 0 85369 644 6
ISBN-13 978 0 85369 644 5

A catalogue record for this book is available from the British Library

To my wife and family

About the author

After qualifying, Alan Nathan was a lecturer in pharmacognosy at Sunderland School of Pharmacy for 2 years, before spending the next 23 years as a community pharmacist, 14 of these as an independent proprietor. In 1989, he was appointed Boots Teacher/Practitioner in the Department of Pharmacy, King's College, London and became a full-time lecturer in pharmacy practice there in 1994. In 2004, he retired from King's College to become a freelance pharmacy writer and consultant.

Alan has published widely in pharmacy and other health profession journals, his main areas of interest being the treatment of minor ailments, and pharmacy law and ethics.

Alan was also a member of the Council of the Royal Pharmaceutical Society from 1986 until 2002, and is co-founder and chairman of the Society's Listening Friends stress help scheme for pharmacists.

Contents

Preface

The first reclassification of a medicine from Prescription-only (POM) to Pharmacy sale (P) status was in 1983. Since then there has been a steady stream of POM-to-P transfers and some 60 medicines are now available over the counter (OTC) that previously could only be obtained by a visit to a doctor. The Government has reaffirmed its commitment to making medicines more accessible to the public and has pledged to continue and increase the rate of POM-to-P reclassifications and, where appropriate, to further deregulate medicines to General sale list (GSL) status to make them even more widely available. The Government has also stated its intention to reclassify medicines for the prevention and treatment of long-term illnesses, and took the first step towards this in 2004 with the licensing of simvastatin for OTC sale for the primary prevention of cardiovascular and cerebrovascular disease.

Pharmacists have traditionally had a major role in the management of minor illness; the importance of this has increased as a result of the POM-to-P reclassification process, and will increase further in the future, broadening with the reclassification of medicines to prevent and treat more serious conditions.

With the advent of nurse prescribing, extended formulary nurse prescribing and supplementary and independent prescribing, other healthcare professionals have also been empowered to authorise supply of non-prescription medicines. These practitioners also need a thorough knowledge of the non-prescription medicines that they can prescribe. Doctors too, although they have knowledge of OTC medicines that were formerly POM, may be unfamiliar with the full range of useful medicines for minor conditions that can be bought in pharmacies and elsewhere.

The usefulness of non-prescription medicines and the important role they play in self-care have tended to be underestimated and the information available about them, including in the main reference sources for medical professionals, is sparse. This book is the only publication in the UK that deals with them comprehensively and in depth. Its aim is to help pharmacists and other healthcare professionals to make well-informed recommendations and prescribing decisions, and assist them to give patients sound advice on non-prescription medicines.

In this book, OTC medicines currently available in the UK are reviewed in alphabetically arranged chapters on the conditions that they are licensed to treat. Information is provided on the following aspects of products and their constituents:

- compounds or constituents
- mode of action
- indications
- evidence of efficacy (see below)
- side-effects
- cautions and contraindications
- interactions
- dosage
- presentations and formulations
- products available and manufacturers (either all products in a category or, for categories where there are a large number of products, a representative selection)
- each section concludes with a summary of key points and suggestions for the most appropriate products to recommend.

Evidence of the efficacy of medicines is cited where it exists. However, very few clinical trials on medicines for OTC use have been published. Most of the available evidence comes from the use of medicines as POMs before their reclassification to P status. In some instances, medicines are licensed for non-prescription use for different indications and at different doses from their use as prescription drugs, and caution may therefore be necessary in extrapolating clinical trial evidence to OTC use. There is very little clinical trial evidence for medicines that were already licensed for OTC use before POM-to-P reclassifications began. Such trials as could be found and appear to meet current methodological standards are cited.

This edition has been completely revised and brought up to date. New products have been included and assessed and discontinued products deleted. New chapters on Fungal nail infection, Migraine and on Cardiovascular medicines for primary and secondary prevention of cardiovascular conditions have been added.

A new feature with this edition is the publication of 6-monthly updates on the Pharmaceutical Press website (www.pharmpress.com/ onlineresources).

Alan Nathan
February 2006

Acne

Acne vulgaris is largely a condition of young people and resolves in the majority of patients by the age of 25 years. It is believed to be nearly universal in adolescents. From a medical point of view, acne vulgaris is a minor problem in most cases. However, its psychological impact on sufferers can be enormous, given that it affects young people at a stage in their lives when they are especially sensitive about their appearance. Patients are often anxious to find a cure for what they consider to be a highly embarrassing problem. About 60% of teenagers consider their condition sufficiently serious to either self-treat with non-prescription products or to seek medical advice. Several effective products for mild-to-moderate acne are available without prescription, although correct use and persistence are necessary to increase the chance of success.

CAUSES

Acne vulgaris is the result of a combination of several factors. The main processes involved are as follows.

- The pilosebaceous units in the dermis of the skin consist of a hair follicle and associated sebaceous glands. These glands secrete sebum – a mixture of fats and waxes – the function of which is to protect the skin and hair by retarding water loss and forming a barrier against external agents. The hair follicle is lined with epithelial cells which become keratinised as they mature.
- During puberty, the production of androgenic hormones increases in both sexes and levels of testosterone rise. Testosterone is taken up into the sebaceous glands, where it is converted into dihydrotestosterone, stimulating the glands to secrete increased amounts of sebum.
- At the same time, the keratin in the follicular epithelial walls becomes unusually cohesive; sebum accumulates within it, forming keratin plugs. These block the openings of the follicles in the epidermis and cause them to dilate beneath the surface of the skin.

- If the orifice of the follicular canal opens sufficiently, the keratinous material is extruded through it and an open comedone results. This is also known as a blackhead because the keratinous material is dark in colour. Because this material can escape, the comedone does not become inflamed. If the follicular orifice does not open sufficiently, a closed comedone (whitehead) results, in which inflammation can occur. Most acne sufferers have a combination of both types of comedone.
- The actions of microorganisms, principally *Propionibacterium acnes*, cause the follicular wall of closed comedones to disrupt and collapse, spilling their contents into the surrounding tissue and provoking an inflammatory response. In addition, bacterial enzymes bring about the decomposition of triglycerides in the sebum to produce free fatty acids, which also cause inflammation. In the more common milder form of acne, this process leads to the formation of papules around the follicular openings; in the more severe form it leads to cyst formation in the deeper layers of the skin.

TREATMENT

Only topical products are available without prescription for the treatment of mild-to-moderate acne. Antibiotics – both systemic and topical – are available on prescription for more severe conditions. The overall aims of topical therapy are to remove follicular plugs, allowing sebum to flow freely, and to minimise bacterial colonisation of the skin. Four main types of preparation are available without prescription:

- keratolytics (also known as comedolytics in relation to acne)
- antimicrobials
- anti-inflammatory agents
- abrasives.

Keratolytics

Compounds available

The compounds available are:

- benzoyl peroxide
- salicylic acid
- sulphur
- resorcinol.

Mode of action

Keratolytic agents promote shedding of the keratinised epithelial cells on the surface of the skin, preventing closure of the pilosebaceous orifice and formation of follicular plugs, and facilitating the flow of sebum. The various compounds cause this effect via different mechanisms. The keratolytic agents also possess varying levels of antimicrobial activity, which contributes to their effectiveness.

Benzoyl peroxide has been in use for the treatment of acne for more than 60 years. It is generally accepted as the most effective topical treatment for mild conditions and there is good evidence to support this.[1-5] There is some difference of opinion over the principal mechanism of action of benzoyl peroxide. It was generally thought that its activity is mainly a comedolytic effect through an irritant action, leading to an increased turnover of the epithelial cells lining the follicular duct and increasing sloughing.[6] More recently, however, its principal mode of action has been suggested to be as a bactericide against *P. acnes*. Benzoyl peroxide is lipophilic and therefore penetrates the follicle well. Once absorbed, it releases oxygen, which suppresses the bacteria, thereby reducing the production of irritant free fatty acids.[7]

Quinoderm (Ferndale) contains potassium hydroxyquinoline sulphate, which has both antibacterial and keratolytic properties, in addition to benzoyl peroxide. A comparison[8] showed this combination to be more effective than benzoyl peroxide alone.

Salicylic acid is used in concentrations of up to 2% for acne. It exerts its keratolytic effect by increasing the hydration of epithelial cells, and it may also have some bacteriostatic activity and a direct anti-inflammatory effect on lesions. It is also believed to enhance penetration into the skin of other medicaments, and is combined with sulphur in some formulary preparations.

Sulphur is claimed to possess keratolytic and antiseptic properties, although this is debatable; it does, however, appear to hasten the resolution of inflammatory pustular lesions.

Some authorities consider preparations based on salicylic acid or sulphur to be obsolete for the treatment of acne, and in the *British National Formulary* they are regarded as a second-line choice. There is little evidence for the effectiveness of salicylic acid in the treatment of acne. Some studies have found proprietary preparations containing salicylic acid to be more effective than benzoyl peroxide, but these studies appear to have been conducted or sponsored by the manufacturer.[9,10]

Resorcinol is only found in combination with sulphur in a single proprietary preparation. It is not regarded as efficacious, has several drawbacks and is not recommended.

Adverse effects, cautions and use

Benzoyl peroxide is mildly irritant and may cause redness, stinging and peeling, especially at the start of treatment, but tolerance usually develops with continued use. To minimise these effects, the lowest available strength (usually 5%) should be used and applied at night for the first week so that any erythema subsides by the next morning. If there is no adverse reaction, application can be twice daily. Several weeks of regular application are usually required to produce real benefit; if the lower strength is ineffective, the higher strength (10%) can be tried. Treatment should not be prolonged beyond 3 months with the 5% preparations or beyond 2 months with the 10% preparations.

True allergy occurs in a very small minority of patients, but allergic contact dermatitis is more common. If troublesome skin irritation occurs, application should be stopped for a day or two; if the same reaction occurs when the product is used again, it should be discontinued. Care should be taken to keep all keratolytics away from the eyes, mouth and other mucous membranes. Benzoyl peroxide is an oxidising agent and may bleach clothing and bedclothes. Concerns were expressed some years ago because animal studies showed that benzoyl peroxide, although not a carcinogen, may promote the growth of tumours.[11] No such fears have been expressed by medicine safety or regulatory bodies in the UK, and benzoyl peroxide is considered safe for human use. A case–control study in England[12] found no significant association between the use of benzoyl peroxide and the occurrence of malignant melanoma.

Salicylic acid is a mild irritant and similar precautions should be adopted as for benzoyl peroxide. Preparations are applied twice or three times a day. Salicylic acid is absorbed readily through the skin and is excreted slowly. Salicylate poisoning can occur if preparations are applied frequently, in large amounts and over large areas.[13] Patients who are sensitive to aspirin should avoid preparations containing salicylic acid.

Resorcinol should not be applied over large areas of skin or for long periods, as it is absorbed and can interfere with thyroid function or cause methaemoglobinaemia. Resorcinol may cause dark-brown scaling on the skin in darker-skinned individuals. Both sulphur and resorcinol can cause skin irritation and sensitisation.

Formulations

Benzoyl peroxide is available in the form of creams, lotions, gels and washes, and in concentrations of 2.5, 5 and 10%. There is little difference in clinical response to the three concentrations in terms of reducing the number of inflammatory lesions, but formulation appears to make a difference.[4] The drying effect of an alcoholic-gel base enhances the effectiveness of the active constituent, and this formulation is more effective than a lotion of the same concentration. However, gels have a greater potential for causing drying of the skin and irritation than preparations in aqueous bland bases. Washes containing benzoyl peroxide have been found to have little or no comedolytic effect, although in a small-scale trial[14] a skin wash containing 2% salicylic acid was found to be more effective than a 10% benzoyl peroxide wash. Brevoxyl (Stiefel) contains 4% benzoyl peroxide formulated in a hydrophase base. The manufacturer claims that the formulation holds the benzoyl peroxide in solution, increasing its bioavailability compared with traditional formulations and preventing the crystallisation of benzoyl peroxide on the skin, which leads to particulate irritation. The manufacturer's own (unpublished) studies show that this formulation is as effective as 10% benzoyl peroxide, but with no more irritant effect than a 2.5% preparation.

Some bases, particularly those of the older formulary products, may reduce the effectiveness of acne products by making the skin more greasy.

Products

- Benzoyl peroxide

  Creams

  — Brevoxyl (4% in hydrophase base)
    Stiefel
  — Oxy On-the-Spot (2.5%)
    Mentholatum
  — PanOxyl 5
    Stiefel
  — Quinoderm cream (10% with 0.5% potassium hydroxyquinoline sulphate)
    Ferndale
  — Quinoderm 5 cream (5% with 0.5% potassium hydroxyquinoline sulphate)
    Ferndale

  Lotions

  — Oxy 10 (10% benzoyl peroxide)
    Mentholatum

Gels

— Acnecide
  Galderma
— PanOxyl 5 Acne Gel (5%)
— PanOxyl 10 Acne Gel (10%)
— PanOxyl Aquagel (2.5%)
  all *Stiefel*

Wash

— PanOxyl Wash 10 (10%)
  Stiefel

- Salicylic acid
  — Acnisal face wash (2%)
    DermaPharm
  — Salicylic Acid and Sulphur Cream BP 1980 (2% salicylic acid and 2% sulphur)
  — Salicylic Acid and Sulphur Ointment BPC 1973 (3% salicylic acid and 3% sulphur)

- Resorcinol
  — Eskamel cream (2% with 8% sulphur)
    Goldshield

Antimicrobials

Compounds available

Compounds available are:

- cetrimide
- chlorhexidine
- povidone-iodine
- triclocarban
- triclosan.

Mode of action

Two of the factors contributing to acne are increased sebum production and *P. acnes*, so a logical approach to treatment is to remove excess sebum from the skin and reduce the bacterial count. To this end, several products containing antibacterial or antiseptic ingredients are available formulated as astringent lotions and detergent-based washes; there are also some antimicrobial creams. There is some evidence to support the effectiveness of antimicrobials. Part of any value of these products may lie in the placebo effect, generated by patients participating in an active routine to deal with their problem.[15,16]

Products

- Cetrimide
  - Torbetol (0.7% with 0.75% chlorhexidine)
    Torbet

- Chlorhexidine
  - Cepton lotion (0.1%)
  - Cepton medicated skin wash (1%)
  - Cepton medicated clear gel (2.5%)
    all *LPC*

- Povidone-iodine
  - Betadine skin cleanser (4%)
    Medlock Medical

- Triclocarban
  - Valderma soap (1%)
    Ransom

- Triclosan
  - Clearasil treatment cream regular (0.1% with 8% sulphur)
    Crookes

Abrasives

Product

There is one product:

- Brasivol No. 1 (fused synthetic aluminium oxide particles in a soap-detergent base)
  Stiefel

Mode of action, use and cautions

This formulation contains small, gritty particles in a skin wash, intended to remove follicular plugs mechanically. However, there is little evidence of the effectiveness of abrasive preparations in acne.[17,18] Recommended use is 1–3 times daily for a duration of 15–20 seconds. The product is contraindicated in the presence of superficial venules or capillaries (telangiectasia), and over-enthusiastic use can cause irritation.

Anti-inflammatory agents

Compounds and products available

Nicotinamide is the only compound available:
- — Freederm Gel (4%)
- — Freederm Lotion (10%)
  both *Dendron*
- — Nicam Gel (4%)
  Dermal

Mode of action and use

Nicotinamide is the physiologically active amide of nicotinic acid and its deficiency in the diet can lead to a range of symptoms, including skin problems. In the topical treatment of acne it is claimed to have anti-inflammatory activity, although its mechanism of action is unknown. It is postulated that nicotinamide might act directly on inflammatory mediators, perhaps through inhibition of neutrophil chemotaxis. In a double-blind clinical trial it was found to be as effective as 1% clindamycin gel in the treatment of mild-to-moderate acne.[19] It does not appear to have been compared directly with benzoyl peroxide. It is applied twice daily. Side-effects include dryness, peeling and irritation similar to those produced by benzoyl peroxide; the same precautions in use should therefore be taken.

PRODUCT SELECTION POINTS

- Benzoyl peroxide is the first-line treatment for mild-to-moderate acne. It has a proven record of efficacy and few drawbacks. A higher strength (10%) formulation of benzoyl peroxide should only be used if 3–4 weeks' treatment with a 5% formulation produces no improvement.
- Alcoholic or astringent gel formulations of benzoyl peroxide are more effective than lotions or creams. However, water-based formulations are less likely to cause skin drying and irritation, and may improve compliance. Washes containing benzoyl peroxide have been found to have little comedolytic effect.
- There is some evidence for the effectiveness of antibacterial preparations.
- All acne treatments must be used regularly for up to 3 months to produce real benefits.

PRODUCT RECOMMENDATIONS

- First choice of treatment for mild-to-moderate acne should be an alcohol- or astringent-based gel containing 5% benzoyl peroxide.
- An aqueous cream or lotion formulation may be preferred by patients with more sensitive skin.

REFERENCES

1. Ozolins M, Eady EA, Avery AJ, *et al*. Comparison of five antimicrobial regimens for treatment of mild to moderate inflammatory facial acne vulgaris in the community: randomised controlled trial. *Lancet* 2004; 64: 2188–2195.
2. Norris JF, Hughes BR, Basey AJ, Cunliffe WJ. A comparison of the effectiveness of topical tetracycline, benzoyl-peroxide gel and oral oxytetracycline in the treatment of acne. *Clin Exp Dermatol* 1991; 16: 31–33.
3. Burke B, Eady EA, Cunliffe WJ. Benzoyl peroxide versus topical erythromycin in the treatment of acne vulgaris. *Br J Dermatol* 1983; 108: 199–204.
4. Mills OH, Kligman AM, Pochi P, Comite H. Comparing 2.5%, 5%, and 10% benzoyl peroxide on inflammatory acne vulgaris. *Int J Dermatol* 1986; 25: 664–667.
5. Lehmann HP, Andrews JS, Robinson KA, *et al*. *Management of acne (Evidence Report/Technology Assessment No 17). Agency for Healthcare Research and Quality Publication No 01-E019*. Rockville, MD: Agency for Healthcare Research and Quality, 2001.
6. Cunliffe WJ, Stainton C, Forster RA. Topical benzoyl peroxide increases the sebum excretion rate in patients with acne. *Br J Dermatol* 1983; 109: 577–579.
7. Bojar RA, Cunliffe WJ, Holland KT. The short-term treatment of acne vulgaris with benzoyl peroxide: effects on the surface and follicular cutaneous microflora. *Br J Dermatol* 1995; 132: 204–208.
8. Jaffe GV, Grimshaw JJ, Constad D. Benzoyl peroxide in the treatment of acne vulgaris: a double-blind, multi-centre comparative study of 'Quinoderm' cream and 'Quinoderm' cream with hydrocortisone versus their base vehicle alone and a benzoyl peroxide only gel preparation. *Curr Med Res Opin* 1989; 11: 453–462.
9. Boutli F, Zioga M, Koussidou T, *et al*. Comparison of chloroxylenol 0.5% plus salicylic acid 2% cream and benzoyl peroxide 5% gel in the treatment of acne vulgaris: a randomized double-blind study. *Drugs Exp Clin Res* 2003; 29: 101–105.

10. Zander E, Weisman S. Treatment of acne vulgaris with salicylic acid pads. *Clin Ther* 1992; 14: 247–253.

11. Jones GRN. Skin cancer: risk to individuals using the tumour promoter benzoyl peroxide for acne treatment. *Hum Toxicol* 1985; 4: 75–78.

12. Cartwright RA, Hughes BR, Cunliffe WJ. Malignant melanoma, benzoyl peroxide and acne: a pilot epidemiological case-control investigation. *Br J Dermatol* 1988; 118: 239–242.

13. Akhavan A, Bershad S. Topical acne drugs: review of clinical properties, systemic exposure, and safety. *Am J Clin Dermatol* 2003; 4: 473–492.

14. Shalita AR. Comparison of a salicylic acid cleanser and a benzoyl peroxide wash in the treatment of acne vulgaris. *Clin Ther* 1989; 11: 264–267.

15. Franz E, Weidner-Strahl S. The effectiveness of topical antibacterials in acne: a double-blind clinical study. *J Int Med Res* 1978; 6:72–77.

16. Stoughton RB, Leyden JJ. Efficacy of 4 percent chlorhexidine gluconate skin cleanser in the treatment of acne vulgaris. *Cutis* 1987; 39: 551–553.

17. Fulghum DD, Catalano PM, Childers RC, *et al*. Abrasive cleansing in the management of acne vulgaris. *Arch Dermatol* 1982; 118: 658–659.

18. Mills OH, Kligman AM. Evaluation of abrasives in acne therapy. *Cutis* 1979; 23: 704–705.

19. Shalita AR, Smith JG, Parish LC, *et al*. Topical nicotinamide compared with clindamycin gel in the treatment of inflammatory acne vulgaris. *Int J Dermatol* 1995; 34: 434–437.

Athlete's foot

Athlete's foot (tinea pedis) is a fungal infection. It most commonly causes itching and weeping between the toes, although other areas of the foot may also be involved.

CAUSES

The causative organisms are a group of fungi known as dermato-phytes, which colonise the horny, outermost layer of the skin. They produce keratinase, which destroys the keratin layer of the epidermis, and also exotoxins, which may cause erythema.

TREATMENT

Preparations for athlete's foot are available in a range of formulations, including ointments, creams, paints, sprays and powders. Powders are usually recommended for dusting into shoes, socks and stockings, either as adjuncts to creams and ointments or to prevent the recurrence of infection once cleared, particularly in individuals who tend to be chronic sufferers. The powder formulation itself helps inhibit the propagation of fungi by adsorbing moisture and preventing skin maceration.

Good foot hygiene is important for effective treatment, and patients should be advised to wash and dry their feet thoroughly before each application of medicament. They should not share towels with others (this helps to prevent the spread of infection), should change their socks, tights or stockings daily, and should be advised to avoid occlusive footwear. It is also important to emphasise the need to apply the medication well beyond the area that can be seen to be infected, and to use it regularly for the full recommended treatment period.

Three groups of drugs are available for the treatment of athlete's foot:

- antifungals
- keratolytic agents
- other antimicrobial compounds, contained in some products.

Antifungals

Compounds available

Compounds available are:

- imidazoles
- terbinafine
- griseofulvin
- tolnaftate
- undecenoates
- benzoic acid.

Mode of action and usage

Terbinafine (an allylamine derivative) and the imidazoles are widely accepted as being the most effective treatments for athlete's foot.[1] They act by inhibiting the biosynthesis of ergosterol, a constituent of the fungal cell membrane, resulting in disruption of the cell. Overall, little difference in efficacy has been found between topical terbinafine and imidazoles in the treatment of fungal infections of the foot, although the former clears infections up to four times more quickly.[2,3]

Imidazoles licensed for treatment of athlete's foot without prescription are clotrimazole, econazole, ketoconazole, miconazole and sulconazole. They are considered to have similar efficacy.[1] These compounds also possess activity against Gram-positive bacteria, which is useful, as secondary bacterial infection may complicate the fungal infection. Application twice or three times daily is recommended, and treatment for at least a month is generally advised to ensure that this tenacious infection is eradicated.

Terbinafine as cream, gel, or spray, is used once or twice daily for 1 week. There is also a single application cutaneous solution that, according to the manufacturer, forms a clear film that releases active ingredient into the skin for up to 13 days. Local irritation and sensitivity are possible with all compounds.

Griseofulvin is an antifungal compound isolated from strains of *Penicillium griseofulvum*. It is exclusively active against dermatophytes through inhibition of cellular mitosis. It also binds to host cell keratin and reduces its degradation by keratinases. It may also interfere with dermatophyte DNA production. A 1% spray solution has been found to be effective against athlete's foot.[4] One spray is applied daily, increasing to three sprays daily for more severe or extensive infection affecting the sides or soles of the feet. Treatment should be continued for 10 days after lesions have disappeared. The treatment period should not exceed 4 weeks.

Tolnaftate is believed to act by distorting fungal hyphae and stunting mycelial growth. It has been shown to be more effective than placebo in the treatment of athlete's foot.[5] It is active against all species responsible for athlete's foot but has no antibacterial activity. It should be used twice daily and treatment should be continued for up to 6 weeks. It is well tolerated when applied to intact or broken skin, although slight stinging on application is probable. Skin reactions are rare and include irritation and contact dermatitis.

Undecenoic acid is an antifungal agent which is effective in chronic cases of mild athlete's foot.[6] Both the acid and its salts are used in proprietary athlete's foot preparations. Undecenoic acid is co-formulated with its zinc salt in one proprietary brand (this is also an official formulary preparation in the United States – Compound Undecylenic Acid Ointment USP). Zinc undecenoate has astringent properties, which helps to reduce the irritation and inflammation caused by the infection. Undecenoic acid, the active antifungal entity, is also liberated from the zinc salt on contact with moisture on the skin. Undecenoic acid and its derivatives are thought to be suitable for mild forms of athlete's foot characterised by dry scaling of tissue, but are less effective where the skin is macerated and moist. Up to 4 weeks' treatment may be needed to produce therapeutic results. Irritation occurs rarely after application of undecenoic acid or its salts. Undecenoic acid and tolnaftate have been found to be equally effective.[7]

Benzoic acid has antifungal activity, lowering the intracellular pH of infecting organisms. It is combined with salicylic acid (a keratolytic agent, see below) in an emulsifying ointment base in Benzoic Acid Ointment, Compound, BP (Whitfield's ointment). This preparation has been in use for over 90 years but more cosmetically acceptable products are now available. The same ingredients in the same proportions are included in Toepedo cream (Dendron). Benzoic acid may cause irritation of the skin, and should not come into contact with the eyes or mucous membranes.

Products

- Terbinafine
  - Lamisil AT (cream, gel and spray)
  - Lamisil Once (single application solution)
    Novartis Consumer Health

- Imidazoles

  Clotrimazole
  - Canesten AF cream, powder and spray
  - Canesten Hydrocortisone cream
    both *Bayer*

  Econazole
  - Ecostatin cream
    Bristol-Myers Squibb
  - Pevaryl cream
    Janssen-Cilag

  Ketoconazole
  - Daktarin Gold cream
    McNeil

  Miconazole
  - Daktarin Dual-action cream, spray powder and powder
  - Daktacort HC cream
    both *McNeil*

- Griseofulvin
  - Grisol AF 1% spray solution
    Transdermal

- Tolnaftate
  - Mycil ointment, powder and spray
    Crookes
  - Tinaderm cream
    Schering-Plough
  - Scholl Athlete's Foot cream, powder, solution and spray
    SSL International

- Undecenoic acid
  - Mycota cream, powder and spray (undecenoic acid/zinc undecenoate)
    SSL International
  - Monphytol paint (contains methyl and propyl undecenoates together with salicylic acid and methyl and propyl salicylates)
    LAB

- Benzoic acid
  - Toepedo cream
    Dendron

Keratolytic agents

Compounds available

Salicylic acid is the only compound available.

Mode of action and usage

Salicylic acid – at concentrations above 2% – has a keratolytic effect, causing the keratin layer of the skin to shed. (Below this concentration it aids normal keratinisation.) Keratolysis is achieved by increasing the hydration of the stratum corneum (the outermost layer of dead cells), softening the cells and facilitating dissolution of the intracellular cement that bonds the cells together so that they separate and detach (desquamate). Moisture is essential to this process and is provided by either the water in the formulation or the occlusive effect produced by its application to the skin. Salicylic acid alone has little or no antifungal activity but it facilitates the penetration of other drugs into the epidermis. Preparations for athlete's foot containing salicylic acid therefore also contain antifungal constituents. Salicylic acid is present at a concentration of 3% in Whitfield's ointment, Toepedo cream and Monphytol paint. Although salicylic acid is readily absorbed through the skin, salicylate poisoning is highly unlikely to result from application to a small area for the limited period of treatment for athlete's foot.

Other antimicrobial compound

Halquinol is a quinoline derivative that possess antibacterial and antifungal activity. It is included at very low concentration as the active constituent of Valpeda cream (Ransom).

PRODUCT SELECTION POINTS

- Terbinafine and imidazole antifungals are generally regarded as first-line treatments. Griseofulvin and tolnaftate have also been shown to be clinically effective, but terbinafine and the imidazoles have additional activity against bacterial supra-infection. Undecenoates appear to be less effective than imidazoles for deeper-seated infections. Other athlete's foot treatments offer no advantage over the above.
- Antifungal powders and sprays may be helpful in preventing recurrence of infection in chronic sufferers.

PRODUCT RECOMMENDATIONS

- First choice of treatment for athlete's foot should be terbinafine or an imidazole antifungal cream. Tolnaftate cream should be used for patients sensitive to these.
- Powders containing the above or undecenoates can be dusted onto the feet and into hosiery and footwear as prophylaxis for chronic sufferers.

REFERENCES

1.   Hart R, Bell-Syer SE, Crawford F, *et al*. Systematic review of topical treatments for fungal infections of the skin and nails of the feet. *BMJ* 1999; 319: 79–82.
2.   Schopf R, Hettler O, Brautigam M, *et al*. Efficacy and tolerability of terbinafine 1% topical solution used for 1 week compared with 4 weeks clotrimazole 1% topical solution in the treatment of interdigital tinea pedis: a randomised controlled clinical trial. *Mycoses* 1999; 42: 415–420.
3.   Leenutaphong V, Tangwiwat S, Muanprasat C, *et al*. Double-blind study of the efficacy of 1 week topical terbinafine cream compared to 4 weeks miconazole cream in patients with tinea pedis. *J Med Assoc Thai* 1999; 82: 1006–1009.
4.   Aly R, Bayles CI, Oakes RA, *et al*. Topical griseofulvin in the treatment of dermatophytoses. *Clin Exp Dermatol* 1994; 19: 43–46.
5.   Tschen EH, Becker LE, Ulrich JA, *et al*. Comparison of over-the-counter agents for tinea pedis. *Cutis* 1979; 23: 696–698.
6.   Chretien JH, Esswein JG, Sharpe LM, *et al*. Efficacy of undecylenic acid-zinc undecylenate powder in culture positive tinea pedis. *Int J Dermatol* 1980; 19: 51–54.
7.   Fuerst JF, Cox GF, Weaver SM, Duncan WC. Comparison between undecylenic acid and tolnaftate in the treatment of tinea pedis. *Cutis* 1980; 25: 544–546.

Cardiovascular medicines

Cardiovascular medicines available without prescription for primary or secondary prevention of cardiovascular disease are:

- simvastatin for reduction of serum cholesterol
- low-dose aspirin for secondary prevention of cerebrovascular as well as cardiovascular disease
- fish oil preparations containing omega-3 fatty acids, which lower serum triglyceride levels.

SIMVASTATIN

Mode of action, efficacy and use

Simvastatin is one of a group of drugs known as statins that act by competitively inhibiting 3-hydroxy-3-methylglutaryl coenzyme A reductase (HMG-CoA reductase), the enzyme that mediates cholesterol synthesis in the liver. Inhibition of HMG-CoA increases the formation of low-density lipoprotein (LDL) receptors on hepatocyte membranes, leading to increased clearance of LDL cholesterol and reduction in total serum cholesterol. While the main biochemical effect of the statins is to lower LDL cholesterol, they also raise levels of high-density lipoprotein (HDL) cholesterol, which improves the HDL:LDL cholesterol ratio (a more important index than total serum cholesterol), and they also reduce plasma triglycerides.

Simvastatin, the first statin to be marketed in the UK, was introduced as a prescription drug in the late 1980s. Simvastatin 10 mg was reclassified for sale without prescription in July 2004, and was the first drug to be made available over the counter (OTC) in the UK for the prevention or treatment of a chronic condition rather than for alleviation of symptoms or treatment of a minor ailment.

Statins have been shown to be safe and effective in lowering cholesterol,[1] and since 2000 it has been recommended that a statin should be prescribed as secondary prevention for all patients with symptomatic cardiovascular disease.[2] More recently, statins have been recommended for all people without symptoms but who are considered to be at 'moderate' (i.e. 10–15% risk of developing coronary heart disease (CHD) within the next 10 years);[3] it is possible to determine moderate risk through self-reported risk factors (see below).[4] However, no specific clinical trials of simvastatin for the specific population for which the drug has been licensed for OTC sale have been carried out, and it has been claimed that the reclassification was not based on robust evidence of clinical benefit or safety.[5]

Indications and licensing restrictions

Simvastatin 10 mg is indicated to reduce the risk of a first major coronary event in individuals at moderate risk of CHD, including:

- men aged 55–70 years, with or without risk factors
- men aged 45–54 years, with one or more listed risk factors
- postmenopausal women aged 55–70 years, with one or more risk factors.

The risk factors are:

- smoker – currently or within the last 5 years
- family history of CHD – father or a brother had a heart attack before 55 years of age, or mother or a sister before 65 years of age
- overweight or obese – body mass index above 25, or waist measurement greater than 40″ (102 cm) in men or greater than 35″ (88 cm) in women
- South-Asian family origin.

Dose

One 10 mg tablet each night, on a long-term basis.

Contraindications and cautions

OTC simvastatin is not suitable for the following groups and in the following circumstances:

- men over 55 years of age with a family history of CHD and at least one other risk factor, as above
- people with, or reporting, any symptoms that might suggest: any cardiovascular, cerebrovascular or peripheral vascular disorder; liver disease or history of abnormal liver function tests; renal impairment; hypothyroidism; myopathy or family history of muscle disorders
- people with a known fasting LDL-cholesterol level of 5.5 mmol/L or above (cholesterol testing before sale is not a licensing requirement but is recommended as good practice by the Royal Pharmaceutical Society of Great Britain [RPSGB])
- people whose blood pressure is known and within the range for referral in accordance with current RPSGB practice guidance (blood pressure testing before sale is not a licensing requirement but is recommended as good practice by the RPSGB)
- men and women who consume more than four or three units of alcohol per day, respectively, and people who drink more than 1 L grapefruit juice per day
- people who have suffered previous side-effects or allergy when taking cholesterol-lowering medication.

These patients should be referred to a doctor.

Adverse effects and interactions

Simvastatin is generally well tolerated and side-effects are usually rare, mild and transient. Myopathy and rhabdomyolysis, characterised by generalised muscle pain, tenderness or weakness, have been reported very rarely. Liver dysfunction, gastrointestinal disturbances and hypersensitivity reactions have also been reported rarely. Drugs that can cause myopathy or rhabdomyolysis, including fibric acid derivatives and nicotinic acid, increase the risk of developing these conditions if given in association with simvastatin.

Simvastatin is metabolised in the liver by the P450 isoenzyme CYP3A4 and interactions can occur with drugs that inhibit this enzyme, including: ciclosporin, itraconazole, ketoconazole, erythromycin, clarithromycin, HIV-protease inhibitors, nefazodone, amiodarone and verapamil. Simvastatin may also increase the anticoagulant effect of warfarin and other coumarins.

Practice guidelines

The RPSGB practice guidance makes the following additional recommendations in association with the OTC sale of simvastatin.

- Pharmacists should be involved in all initial sales but subsequent sales may be delegated to appropriately trained medicines counter assistants.
- Where possible, sales should be recorded in the patient's medication record.
- Life-style advice to reduce the risk of CHD should be given to purchasers.
- Pharmacists should liaise with local doctors and primary-care organisation to fit in with local policies on management of CHD risk and prescribing of statins; they should encourage purchasers to inform their doctor that they are taking simvastatin.
- Pharmacists should monitor people who buy simvastatin at least once a year for adverse effects, interactions, changes in risk factors and blood cholesterol levels.

Product

- Zocor Heart-Pro
  McNeil

ASPIRIN (ANTIPLATELET)

Mode of action

Low-dose aspirin reduces the risk of myocardial infarction (MI), increases survival in patients who have had an acute MI and reduces the risk of stroke, through inhibiting thrombus formation within coronary and cerebral blood vessels. The anti-inflammatory and anti-thrombotic effects of aspirin depend on its ability to inactivate the enzyme cyclo-oxygenase. Platelets (thrombocytes) in the blood play an important role in the process of coagulation. Through irreversible inhibition of cyclo-oxygenase, aspirin prevents the synthesis of thromboxane A_2 which promotes platelet adhesion and aggregation. Platelets cannot synthesise more thromboxane A_2, which is restored only when existing platelets are replaced from the vascular endothelium. Continuous low dosing with aspirin thereby maintains thromboxane A_2 at a low level. Systematic reviews have confirmed that aspirin at a daily dose of 75–325 mg is effective for the secondary prevention of serious vascular events and reduces all-cause mortality.[6,7]

Uses

Low-dose aspirin is indicated for the secondary prevention of thrombotic cerebrovascular and cardiovascular disease, at a dose of 75 mg daily. A single dose of 150–300 mg is also given as emergency first aid to someone who is suspected to have suffered an MI or stroke whilst awaiting the attendance of medical personnel. Low-dose aspirin is also indicated for primary prevention of MI or stroke when the estimated 10-year cardiovascular disease risk is 20% or greater.

Antiplatelet aspirin therapy should only be initiated on the advice of a doctor. The same contraindications, cautions and interactions apply as for aspirin at analgesic doses (see chapter on Pain).

Products

Generic products

Aspirin, 75 mg, is available as standard, dispersible and enteric-coated tablets. For generic products, legal classification, availability and maximum amount that may be supplied in a single sale depends on formulation and pack size see the table below.

Generic aspirin 75 mg tablets: legal classification, availability and maximum amount that may be supplied in a single sale

Formulation	Pack size	Legal status	Availability	Maximum supply
Standard	Up to 16	GSL	Any retail outlet	100
	17–100	GSL	Pharmacy only	100
Dispersible	Up to 30	GSL	Any retail outlet	No limit
	> 30	GSL	Pharmacy only	No limit
Enteric coated	Up to 28	GSL	Any retail outlet	100
	Up to 100	P	Pharmacy	100

GSL, General sale list; P, Pharmacy medicine.

Proprietary products

All the brands below have Pharmacy medicine status.

- Standard tablets
  - — Angettes 75
    Bristol-Myers Squibb

- Dispersible tablets
  - — Pure Health
    Lexon

- Enteric-coated tablets
  - — Caprin 75 mg
    Pinewood

— Micropirin
  Ratiopharm
— Nu-seals 75
  Alliance

OMEGA-3 TRIGLYCERIDES

Mode of action and use

Omega-3 triglycerides are derived from fish oils. They contain triglycerides of omega-3 fatty acids, particularly eicosapentaenoic acid (EPA) and docosahexaenoic acid (DHA). These exert an antithrombotic effect by competing with arachidonic acid for inclusion in cyclo-oxygenase and lipoxygenase synthesis pathways, reducing platelet aggregation and decreasing platelet counts. They also lower blood cholesterol levels through reduction of very-low-density-lipoproteins. As cyclo-oxygenase inhibitors they also have anti-inflammatory activity.

A systematic review[8] has concluded that EPA and DHA in fish oil have a role in the secondary prevention of cardiovascular disease, clinical trial data having demonstrated a significant reduction in total mortality, death from CHD and sudden death in patients taking these oils.

Products

Many products containing fish oils are available as food supplements. One Pharmacy medicine, Omacor (Solvay), is licensed for use in secondary prevention following MI and for the treatment of hyper-triglyceridaemia. Maxepa (Seven Seas) is licensed for the treatment of hypertriglyceridaemia.

REFERENCES

1. Baigent C, Keech A, Kearney PM, *et al*; Cholesterol Treatment Trialists' (CTT) Collaborators. Efficacy and safety of cholesterol-lowering treatment: prospective meta-analysis of data from 90,056 participants in 14 randomised trials of statins. *Lancet* 2005; 366: 1267–1278.
2. Department of Health. *Coronary Heart Disease: National Service Framework for Coronary Heart Disease. Modern standards and service models.* London: HMSO: 2000.
3. Williams B, Poulter NR, Brown MJ, *et al*; British Hypertension Society. Guidelines for management of hypertension: report of the fourth working party of the British Hypertension Society, 2004–BHS IV. *J Hum Hypertens* 2004; 18: 139–185.
4. Royal Pharmaceutical Society of Great Britain. *Practice Guidance: OTC Simvastatin.* London: RPSGB, 2004.
5. Simvastatin over the counter. *Drug Ther Bull* 2005; 43: 25–28.
6. Antithrombotic Trialists' Collaboration. Collaborative meta-analysis of randomised trials of antiplatelet therapy for prevention of death, myocardial infarction and stroke in high risk patients. *BMJ* 2002; 324: 71–86.
7. Weisman SM, Graham DY. Evaluation of the benefits and risks of low-dose aspirin in the secondary prevention of cardiovascular and cerebrovascular events. *Arch Intern Med* 2002; 162: 2197–2202.
8. Harper CR, Jacobson TA. Usefulness of omega-3 fatty acids and the prevention of coronary heart disease. *Am J Cardiol* 2005; 96: 1521–1529.

Colds

Colds normally present as a complex or sequence of symptoms. Products marketed for their treatment usually contain several ingredients, each intended to alleviate a different symptom. As is frequently the case with self-treatment, the psychologically beneficial effect on the sufferer of doing something to relieve the discomfort caused by the cold, plus the expectations raised by advertising or recommendation, may be as important as the intrinsic therapeutic properties of a product's ingredients. Although it is probably better to recommend individual medicines in response to specific symptoms, the public seems to prefer 'all-in-one' remedies and these often cost less than two or three separate products.

CAUSES

Patients frequently confuse colds and influenza, self-diagnosing 'flu' when they have a heavy cold. However, the two conditions are caused by different viruses and influenza is a more serious infection. Indeed, patients who have genuine influenza are usually too ill to get out of bed, and would not present in the pharmacy for advice and treatment but would have to send a representative.

As long as there are no complications, treatment is symptomatic and essentially the same for both conditions.

A common cold usually begins with a sensation of smarting or tingling in the nose, throat and possibly eyes, and progresses to sneezing and rhinorrhoea (runny nose). Inflammation and swelling of the mucosae of the nasal passages may then occur, leading to congestion (blocked nose, stuffiness). The throat often also becomes inflamed, causing soreness and possibly reflex coughing, which may also be provoked by mucus dripping down from the nasopharynx into the bronchus (postnasal drip). In children, a raised temperature may accompany a common cold.

Cold remedies mostly contain constituents intended to relieve one or more of the symptoms described above. They also often include analgesics/antipyretics, although raised temperature and muscular pains are not usual features of the common cold in adults, but are characteristic of influenza.

Most systemic products for colds contain combinations of two or more of the following:

- sedating antihistamine
- sympathomimetic decongestant
- expectorant
- cough suppressant
- analgesic/antipyretic.

The last three groups of ingredients are described in some detail in the chapters on Cough and Pain and only additional information relating specifically to their inclusion in cold remedies is given here.

In addition, a number of volatile substances are included in products to be inhaled for the relief of cold symptoms.

Antihistamines

One of the antimuscarinic side-effects of sedating antihistamines – the drying up of nasal secretions – is exploited in cold remedies to counteract rhinorrhoea. The suppression of rhinorrhoea in turn provokes congestion, however, and antihistamines are usually co-formulated with sympathomimetics to offset this effect. There is no evidence that any antihistamine is preferable to another in the treatment of rhinorrhoea. Sympathomimetics may also help to counteract the sedation caused by antihistamines, but not other side-effects such as dry mouth, urinary retention and blurred vision. Two systematic reviews[1,2] have concluded that antihistamines alone are of little clinical benefit in colds, but that antihistamine–decongestant combinations have a beneficial effect on general recovery as well as on nasal symptoms, in adults and older children. It is, however, not clear whether these effects are clinically significant.

Product examples

Antihistamines are formulated with sympathomimetic decongestants in the following products:

- Benylin 4-Flu liquid and tablets (diphenhydramine/ pseudoephedrine)
  Pfizer Consumer Healthcare

- Multi-Action Actifed syrup and tablets (triprolidine/ pseudoephedrine)
  Pfizer Consumer Healthcare

- Vicks Medinite (doxylamine/pseudoephedrine)
  Procter & Gamble

Systemic decongestants

Decongestants are included in cold remedies to constrict the swollen mucosae and dilated blood vessels of the nasal passages in order to improve air circulation and mucus drainage. The same compounds are used as in cough preparations (see chapter on Cough), plus phenylephrine, although this drug is not considered to be effective orally because of irregular absorption and first-pass metabolism in the liver. Phenylephrine is the only systemic decongestant licensed for use in General sale list products.

Local decongestants

Compounds employed for local use exert a rapid and potent vaso-constricting effect when applied directly to the affected tissue.

Compounds available

The following compounds are available:

- ephedrine
- oxymetazoline
- phenylephrine
- xylometazoline.

Mode of action and cautions

When used topically inside the nose, the vasoconstricting action of sympathomimetic decongestants prevents their absorption, thereby confining activity to the area of application. They can therefore generally be used by patients for whom systemic decongestants are contraindicated. Although the likelihood of interactions is low, patients taking monoamine oxidase inhibitors should not use topical decongestants.

Topical sympathomimetic decongestants have a rapid and potent action. Their disadvantage is that, if used for prolonged periods, they cause a rebound effect (rebound congestion, also known as secondary hyperaemia or rhinitis medicamentosa), with the congestion returning, often worse than before. This is thought to be the result of compensatory vasodilatation as the tissues become conditioned to the drug and its effects wear off. A systematic review[3] found that, in the common cold, a single dose of nasal decongestant, either oral or topical, is moderately effective for the short-term relief of congestion in adults, but there is no evidence to show benefit over a longer period. It also found insufficient data on the use of these medications in children and therefore could not recommend their use in young children with the common cold.

The longer-acting compounds, xylometazoline and oxymetazoline, take longer to produce rebound congestion than the shorter-acting ephedrine and phenylephrine. Dosing is also more convenient with longer-acting compounds, as they are effective for up to 12 hours and thus only need to be used twice or three times daily compared with every 3–4 hours for the shorter-acting compounds. To prevent rebound congestion, the shorter-acting topical decongestants should not be used for more than 5 days or the longer-acting compounds for more than 7 days. Rebound congestion does not occur when sympathomimetic decongestants are taken orally.

Product presentation

Topical decongestants are available as sprays or drops. Sprays are preferable for adults and older children, as a fine mist provides better distribution of medicament around the area of application. Drops are more likely to be swallowed and absorbed systemically but greater ease of application makes them more suitable for children under 6 years of age.

Product examples

Products available include:

- Ephedrine
    - Ephedrine Nasal Drops BP (0.5%)

- Oxymetazoline spray (0.05%)
    - Afrazine
      Schering-Plough
    - Vicks Sinex Decongestant Nasal Spray and Micro Mist
      Procter & Gamble

- Phenylephrine
    - Fenox drops and spray (0.5%)
      Thornton & Ross

- Xylometazoline
    — Otrivine adult formula drops (0.1%) and Otrivine
      children's formula drops (0.05%)
    — Otrivine measured-dose sinusitis spray and Otrivine adult
      menthol nasal spray (both 0.1%)
      all *Novartis Consumer Health*
    — Sudafed decongestant spray (0.1%)
      Pfizer Consumer Healthcare

Inhalants

A wide variety of volatile substances are included in products
intended to be inhaled, either directly or via steam inhalations, for the
relief of cold symptoms. They all have a pungent, aromatic odour.
There is no objective evidence that they improve cold symptoms, but
products containing these substances have been popular for generations and they undeniably produce a temporary sensation of clearing the nasal passages.

In theory, at least, use of volatile products in steam inhalations
should be helpful as the steam itself could be expected to liquefy
mucus secretions and make removal easier. A Cochrane Review[4] sup-
ports the use of warm vapour inhalations for relief of symptoms of
the common cold. Excessive use of inhalants without steam may make
matters worse, however, through reducing clearance of mucus by
impairing the action of cilia in the upper respiratory tract.

Constituents and presentation

Inhalant preparations contain 2–6 volatile ingredients, combinations
differing between products. There is little information available about
their action on respiratory tract tissue, and their use appears to be
empirical and based on tradition. The most frequently included constituent is menthol, and other popular ingredients are eucalyptus oil,
benzoin, camphor, methyl salicylate, thymol, pine oil and peppermint

oil. Creosote, clove oil, aniseed oil, juniper berry oil, turpentine oil, cajuput oil, terpineol, chlorbutol and chlorocresol are also included in some products. Concentrations of constituents vary widely between products.

Nearly all ingredients of inhalant products have a counterirritant effect when applied locally. Thymol, chlorbutol and chlorocresol are phenolic antiseptics with antibacterial and antifungal activity, although their inclusion in inhalant preparations would seem to be for their strong 'medicinal' aroma.

Inhalants are presented as steam inhalations (e.g. Menthol and Eucalyptus Inhalation BP 1980), oils that can be inhaled directly or via steam inhalations (e.g. Karvol capsules and drops [Crookes]; Olbas Oil [GR Lane] and salves to be applied around the throat and upper chest or used in steam inhalations (e.g. Snufflebabe [Pickles]; Vicks VapoRub [Procter & Gamble] ; Mentholatum vapour rub [Mentholatum]). Volatile substances are also presented as pastilles to be sucked (e.g. Potter's Catarrh Pastilles [Ernest Jackson]) and solid stick inhalants (e.g. Vicks Inhaler). The fairly complicated procedure involved in steam inhalations may well improve the efficacy of any product used through an attention-placebo effect.

Vitamin C

Several compound cold treatments contain vitamin C in the range 40–300 mg per dose. The use of this vitamin in the treatment of the common cold has been the subject of debate for more than 30 years, since 'mega doses' were first advocated as both prophylaxis and cure.[5] Current opinion from systematic reviews is that vitamin C supplementation does not reduce the incidence of colds in the normal population and that routine mega-dose prophylaxis or taking vitamin C at the first sign of a cold is not effective, although regular intake of vitamin C may slightly reduce the duration of cold symptoms.[6,7]

Taking mega doses of vitamin C can have adverse consequences, particularly for groups of patients who are already at risk. Vitamin C is a reducing agent and may interfere with diabetic urine glucose tests.

It has also been reported to counteract the action of anticoagulants, and it may increase the production of urinary oxalate, leading to renal stones. The adverse effect likely to be of greatest relevance to community pharmacists results from the formulation of high doses of vitamin C as effervescent tablets. Large quantities of sodium bicarbonate are required in this formulation, which could disturb the electrolyte balance of patients with cardiovascular conditions, especially those whose sodium intake is restricted.

PRODUCT SELECTION POINTS

- Although, from a clinical point of view, it is preferable to recommend individual products in response to specific cold symptoms, patients tend to find combination products more convenient, and these often work out cheaper than two or three individual medicines.
- Local sympathomimetic decongestants (drops or sprays) can generally be used by patients in whom systemic decongestants are contraindicated.
- The longer-acting local sympathomimetic decongestants, oxymetazoline and xylometazoline, are preferable to shorter-acting compounds, as less frequent application is needed and they can be used for slightly longer periods without risk of rebound congestion.
- For adults, spray presentations of local decongestants are preferable to drops, but sprays should not be used in children under 6 years of age.
- Although there is no objective proof that volatile inhalants improve cold symptoms, they enjoy a long-standing popularity and are safe to use in patients of all ages (the proprietary products have different minimum ages) and in all risk groups.

PRODUCT RECOMMENDATIONS

There is little evidence of the effectiveness for some products for colds and 'flu', and others might be regarded as examples of inappropriate polypharmacy. Nevertheless, two factors create a strong demand for these: the desire of sufferers to alleviate their symptoms and their willingness to try anything that might bring relief, and the expectations created by advertising. Thus, while 'all-in-one' night-time cold treatments or antihistamine/decongestant combinations might not accord with the principles of rational product selection, there is a strong demand for them.

Some formulations can, however, be recommended with confidence that they are rational and normally effective choices, while others will provide some symptomatic relief and are harmless. These include:

- for colds and 'flu' with nasal congestion (in normal healthy adults) – analgesics/antipyretics combined with sympathomimetic decongestants, either paracetamol/pseudoephedrine (e.g. Non-Drowsy Sinutab Tablets [Pfizer Consumer Healthcare] and other brands) or ibuprofen/pseudoephedrine (e.g. Nurofen Cold and Flu Tablets [Crookes] and other brands). Some decongestant/analgesic combinations are available as powders to prepare hot drinks (e.g. Lemsip Max Flu Lemon [Reckitt Benckiser]); the making of a hot drink may add to any placebo effect.
- For nasal congestion – decongestant nasal sprays (drops for children), such as xylometazoline.
- As inhalations – Menthol and Eucalyptus Inhalation; but inhalant oils (e.g. Karvol capsules [Crookes], Olbas Oil [GR Lane] and salves (e.g. Vicks VapoRub [Procter & Gamble]) may be preferred for convenience.

REFERENCES

1. De Sutter AIM, Lemiengre M, Campbell H, Mackinnon HF. Antihistamines for the common cold. *The Cochrane Library*, issue 3. Chichester, UK: John Wiley & Sons, 2003 (www.thecochranelibrary.com).
2. D'Agostino RB, Weintraub M, Russell HK, *et al*. The effectiveness of antihistamines in reducing the severity of runny nose and sneezing: a meta-analysis. *Clin Pharmacol Ther* 1998; 64: 579–596.
3. Taverner D, Bickford L, Draper M. Nasal decongestants for the common cold. *The Cochrane Library*, issue 2. Chichester, UK: John Wiley & Sons, 2004 (www.thecochranelibrary.com).
4. Singh M. Heated, humidified air for the common cold. *The Cochrane Library*, issue 2. Chichester, UK: John Wiley & Sons, 2004 (www.the cochranelibrary.com).
5. Pauling L. *Vitamin C and the Common Cold*. San Francisco: WH Freeman, 1976.
6. Hemilä H, Chalker E, D'Souza RRD, *et al*. Vitamin C for preventing and treating the common cold. *The Cochrane Library*, issue 4. Chichester, UK: John Wiley & Sons, 2004 (www.thecochranelibrary.com).
7. Douglas R, Hemila H. Vitamin C for preventing and treating the common cold. *PLoS Medicine* 2005; 2: 132–133.

Cold sores

Cold sores (herpes simplex labialis) are a recurrent infection of the area around the lips and mouth.

CAUSES

Cold sores are caused by the herpes simplex virus type 1 (HSV-1). They are very common – about 80% of the population are asymptomatic carriers of the virus, and 20–25% of these (about 8 million people) suffer, on average, two symptomatic outbreaks per year. Once contracted, HSV-1 is never eliminated from the body. Following the attacks, it regresses to the ganglia of the trigeminal and lumbosacral nerves, where it lies dormant until one of several trigger factors or lowered immunity allows it to break out again. Cold sores frequently occur in association with the common cold, hence the name. The condition also often follows exposure to the sun, giving rise to its other common name, sun blisters.

Outbreaks follow a characteristic pattern, with a prodromal phase of up to 24 hours before any visible signs appear, during which the area on or around the lips begins to tingle, burn or itch. Erythema then develops, followed by the formation of painful and irritating fluid-filled blisters, which break down into shallow, weeping ulcers. The ulcers then dry and form crusts, which are shed, and the area heals within about 7 days. The total length of an episode is usually 10–20 days.

TREATMENT

Cold sores are difficult to treat – even systemic antiviral therapy has not proven particularly effective.[1,2] A number of topical non-prescription products are available:

- antiviral agents: aciclovir and penciclovir
- antiseptics, astringents and local anaesthetics – intended to alleviate symptoms.

Aciclovir

Mode of action

Aciclovir is a synthetic analogue of guanine. Its spectrum of activity is specific to human pathogenic viruses that produce thymidine kinase, of which HSV-1 is one. The activity of aciclovir depends on its conversion by thymidine kinase within infected cells to aciclovir monophosphate, which is then converted by cellular enzymes to aciclovir triphosphate. Aciclovir triphosphate is incorporated by virus-specific DNA polymerase into viral DNA instead of the deoxyguanosine triphosphate required for DNA synthesis and replication. The DNA chain is thereby terminated and replication cannot occur. Aciclovir also inhibits the virus-specific DNA polymerase by acting as a 'decoy' substrate.

Use and efficacy

The manufacturers recommend that aciclovir cream should be used as soon as prodromal symptoms occur, to prevent progress of the cold sore, either stopping it altogether or limiting the severity of the attack. The cream should be applied five times daily, at 4-hourly intervals, but omitting an application in the middle of the night; treatment should be continued for 5 days. If healing is not complete after this time, treatment can be continued for a further 5 days. Patients should be referred to a doctor if lesions are not healed within 3 weeks.

There is equivocal evidence of the effectiveness of topical aciclovir as a treatment for cold sores. Several clinical trials have shown little or no benefit of aciclovir over placebo in reduction of pain or itching, and little or no effect on shortening the duration of the infection if the product is used after lesions have appeared.[3–5] Some trials have demonstrated a reduction in the median time to healing of 1 or 2 days if the cream is used from the first onset of prodromal symptoms, although the severity of symptoms was not reduced.[6] In one trial, lesions did not progress beyond the erythema stage in a small proportion of subjects treated with aciclovir, compared with none in the placebo group.[7] Another trial found aciclovir cream to have no clinical advantage over placebo, although both were better than no treatment.[8]

It has been suggested that use of aciclovir cream may reduce the length of subsequent cold sore attacks by reducing the reservoir of virus in the nerve ganglia, although there is no evidence from clinical trials for this.

There is limited evidence that aciclovir cream has prophylactic action against the recurrence of cold sores, but little proof that it protects against attacks caused by ultraviolet radiation, one of the most common triggers of the condition, although high-factor sunscreens have been found to provide effective protection.[1,9]

Adverse effects and cautions

Transient burning and stinging may occur following application, and a small proportion of patients experience erythema, itching or mild drying or flaking of the skin. Care should be taken not to get cream inside the mouth or in the eyes, as it is irritant to mucous membranes. (Particular care should be taken by all patients with cold sores not to touch their eyes, as transfer of the virus can cause herpes keratitis, a serious and potentially sight-threatening infection.)

Aciclovir cream is licensed for use in children and pregnant women, and is only contraindicated in patients hypersensitive to the antiviral itself, or to propylene glycol, which is contained in the base.

Products

Several brands of aciclovir 5% cream are licensed for non-prescription sale.

Penciclovir

A consultation was issued by the MHRA in January 2006 on an application to reclassify penciclovir 1% cream to pharmacy status, with the proprietary name of Fenistil (Novartis Consumer Health).

By the time of going to press this product had not been marketed. Progress will be reported via the 6-monthly updates on the Pharmaceutical Press website (see Preface).

Penciclovir is structurally related to aciclovir and has a similar mechanism of action. Clinical trials have shown that penciclovir is as effective or superior to aciclovir in the treatment of herpes labialis.[4,10,11] It requires application at 2-hourly intervals during waking hours and treatment should be continued for 4 days.

It is not licensed for use in children under 12 years or for pregnant or breastfeeding women. Otherwise adverse effects and cautions are as for aciclovir cream.

Other treatments

Compound preparations containing antimicrobial, local anaesthetic, counterirritant and astringent constituents in various combinations are available.

Mode of action

As cold sores are uncomfortable and often painful, but self-limiting, the principal aim of treatment is to reduce discomfort while the infection takes its course. Constituents with local anaesthetic and analgesic effects, such as lidocaine, choline salicylate and phenol, are included for this purpose. Counterirritants such as ammonia solution and menthol produce sensations of warmth and coolness, respectively, and may mask discomfort. The bland cream bases of some products may also have a soothing effect.

Astringents such as zinc sulphate and tannic acid precipitate proteins in the lesions, and are presumably included to promote faster healing, although there is no evidence that they do this. Lotions and gels with alcoholic bases may also be employed to accelerate healing as they have a drying effect on the sores. Antimicrobials are presumably included to prevent secondary bacterial infections from complicating and prolonging attacks, although this rarely occurs.

Combination preparations for cold sores are relatively innocuous, although repeated use of local anaesthetics can cause sensitisation. The cream formulations can be applied as frequently as necessary; the use of lotion and gel formulations is, however, limited to three or four applications per day.

Products

- **Blistex Relief Cream** (strong ammonia solution, aromatic ammonia solution and phenol)
  Dendron

- **Bonjela Gel** (choline salicylate and cetalkonium chloride; can also be used in the treatment of mouth ulcers – see chapter on Mouth ulcers)
  Reckitt Benckiser

- **Colsor cream and lotion** (tannic acid, phenol and menthol)
  Ransom

- **Cymex cream** (urea, cetrimide, chlorocresol and dimeticone)
  EC De Witt

- **Lypsyl Cold Sore Gel** (lidocaine, zinc sulphate and cetrimide)
  Novartis Consumer Health

PRODUCT SELECTION POINTS

- Aciclovir cream appears to have little effect on cold sore symptoms, but may reduce the length of an attack if used as soon as prodromal symptoms begin.
- Combination preparations are unlikely to shorten attacks but they contain constituents that may provide symptomatic relief.
- Aciclovir and penciclovir creams are considerably more expensive than the combination products, and it is therefore probably more cost-effective for people who suffer cold sores only

occasionally to use the latter. Chronic sufferers may find it useful to keep aciclovir or penciclovir cream ready to use at the first sign of an attack.

- For sufferers whose attacks are triggered by sunlight, an ultra-violet-blocking lip salve or high-factor sunscreen is an effective prophylactic.

PRODUCT RECOMMENDATIONS

- For occasional sufferers – a combination product containing analgesic ingredients.
- For chronic sufferers to have ready to use at the onset of pro-dromal symptoms – aciclovir cream.
- As prophylaxis against sun blisters – a sun-blocking lip salve or high-factor sunscreen.

REFERENCES

1. Worrall G. Herpes labialis. *Clin Evid* 2004; 11: 2174–2181.
2. Jensen LA, Hoehns JD, Squires CL. Oral antivirals for the acute treatment of recurrent herpes labialis. *Ann Pharmacother* 2004; 38: 705–709.
3. Spruance SL, Nett R, Marbury T, *et al*. Acyclovir cream for treatment of herpes simplex labialis: results of two randomized, double-blind, vehicle-controlled, multicenter clinical trials. *Antimicrob Agents Chemother* 2002; 46: 2238–2243.
4. Femiano F, Gombos F, Scully C. Recurrent herpes labialis: efficacy of topical therapy with penciclovir compared with acyclovir (aciclovir). *Oral Dis* 2001; 7: 31–33.
5. Raborn GW, McGaw WT, Grace M, Houle L. Herpes labialis treatment with acyclovir 5 per cent ointment. *J Can Dent Assoc* 1989; 55: 135–137.
6. Van Vloten WA, Swart RN, Pot F. Topical acyclovir therapy in patients with recurrent orofacial herpes simplex infections. *J Antimicrob Chemother* 1983; 12 Suppl B: 89–93.
7. Fiddian AP, Yeo JM, Stubbings R, Dean D. Successful treatment of herpes labialis with topical acyclovir. *BMJ (Clin Res Ed)* 1983; 286: 1699–1701.
8. Shaw M, King M, Best JM, Banatvala JE, *et al*. Failure of acyclovir cream in treatment of recurrent herpes labialis. *BMJ (Clin Res Ed)* 1985; 291: 7–9.
9. Rooney JF, Bryson Y, Mannix ML, *et al*. Prevention of ultraviolet-light-induced herpes labialis by sunscreen. *Lancet* 1991; 338: 1419–1422.

10. Lin L, Chen XS, Cui PG, *et al*. Topical Penciclovir Clinical Study Group. Topical application of penciclovir cream for the treatment of herpes simplex facialis/labialis: a randomized, double-blind, multicentre, aciclovir-controlled trial. *J Dermatol Treat* 2002; 13: 67–72.

11. Raborn GW, Martel AY, Lassonde M, *et al*; Worldwide Topical Penciclovir Collaborative Study Group. Effective treatment of herpes simplex labialis with penciclovir cream: combined results of two trials. *J Am Dent Assoc* 2002; 133: 303–309.

Constipation

(continued . . .)

Constipation that is not secondary to underlying disease or caused by factors such as side-effects of drugs or laxative abuse is known as simple or functional constipation and may be self-treated on the basis of advice from a pharmacist.

CAUSES

Simple constipation has various causes but may be caused by insufficient fluid and fibre in the diet, resulting in low stool volume. Bowel evacuation is inhibited because of the consequent lack of stimulus of peristalsis in the colon. Correcting such dietary deficiencies often resolves the problem, although patients do not always appreciate that time is needed for such changes to take effect. Some patients are unable to take dietary measures or find them unsuccessful; laxatives may be a useful short-term measure in these cases.

TREATMENT

Laxatives can be broadly classified into five groups depending on their mode of action:

- bulk-forming laxatives
- stimulant laxatives
- osmotic laxatives
- faecal softeners
- faecal lubricants.

Several products are also available for use as bowel evacuants prior to abdominal investigation procedures. Although these can be sold without prescription, they should be used only under medical direction and are not discussed here.

The efficacy of laxatives is surprisingly little researched, and much of the existing work is on elderly subjects. Some systematic reviews and meta-analyses have been published, and these generally conclude that there is evidence of effectiveness for most laxatives; however, there is little evidence available as to their comparative effectiveness.[1-4]

Bulk-forming laxatives

Constituents

Bulk-forming laxatives contain one of the following:

- ispaghula husk
- sterculia
- methylcellulose.

Mode of action

Bulk-forming laxatives provide the closest approximation to the natural process of increasing faecal volume, and are the first-line recommendation for functional constipation. They contain natural or semi-synthetic polysaccharides or cellulose derivatives that pass through the gastrointestinal tract undigested. They increase faecal volume through three mechanisms, the relative contribution of each depending on the composition and properties of the substance. The first action is to add directly to the volume of the intestinal contents. Ispaghula husk (which consists of the seed coats of various species of plantago, a plantain) and sterculia (also known as Indian tragacanth or karaya gum, a gum from the tropical shrub *Sterculia urens*) contain mucilloid constituents that bind water and swell in the colonic lumen to form a gel, thereby softening the faeces and increasing their bulk. Methylcellulose is a semi-synthetic hydrophilic colloid with a similar action. Bulk laxatives also add to faecal mass by acting as substrates for the growth of colonic bacteria. There appears to have been no comparison of the effectiveness of bulk-forming laxatives. Some patients may find some preparations more palatable than others.

Dosage and administration

- **Ispaghula:** adults, one sachet (Fybogel, Konsyl, Regulan) or two teaspoonfuls (Isogel) twice daily; children 6–12 years, half adult dose. The preparation should be stirred into about 150 mL of cold water and taken immediately, preferably after meals.
- **Sterculia** (Normacol, Normacol Plus): adults, one or two heaped 5 mL spoonfuls or one or two sachets once or twice daily after meals; children 6–12 years (Normacol only; Normacol Plus not recommended), half adult dose. The granules should be placed on the tongue and washed down, without chewing, with plenty of water.
- **Methylcellulose:** adults, three to six 500 mg tablets (Celevac) twice daily, swallowed with at least 300 mL of water.

None of the above preparations should be taken immediately before going to bed, because there may be a risk (which is more likely with water-insoluble fibre products) of oesophageal blockage if the patient lies down directly after taking them. As bulk laxatives have a natural action, patients should be warned not to expect an immediate effect. They usually act within 24 hours, but 2–3 days of medication may be required to achieve a full effect.

Cautions and contraindications

As bulk-forming laxatives are not absorbed, they have no systemic effects; also, they do not interact with other medicines and do not appear to interfere significantly with drug absorption. However, there is a risk of oesophageal and intestinal obstruction if preparations are not taken with plenty of water. It is therefore important to stress the importance of following instructions for administration carefully.

Abdominal distension and flatulence are possible side-effects, and for this reason bulk-forming laxatives may cause discomfort if taken in the later stages of pregnancy. They are not contraindicated in pregnancy, although the general precautions that apply to use of any medicine should be observed.

Some bulk-forming laxative preparations contain glucose, which should be taken into account when making recommendations for patients with diabetes. Bulk laxatives may not be suitable for patients who need to restrict their fluid intake severely.

Products

- Ispaghula husk (also known as plantago or psyllium)
  — Isogel granules
    Chefaro UK
  — Ispagel sachets
    LPC
  — Manevac granules (also contains senna)
    Galen
  — Regulan sachets
    Procter & Gamble
  — Senokot Hi-Fibre sachets
    Reckitt Benckiser

- Sterculia
  — Normacol granules and sachets; Normacol Plus granules and sachets (also contain frangula)
    Norgine

- Methylcellulose
  — Celevac tablets
    Shire

Stimulant laxatives

Mode of action and use

The effect of stimulant laxatives is thought to be produced mainly by stimulation of the intestinal mucosa to secrete water and electrolytes. This is achieved through one or both of two possible mechanisms. The first is inhibition of the sodium pump (the enzyme sodium–potassium adenosine triphosphatase [Na$^+$/K$^+$ ATPase]), which prevents sodium transport across the intestinal wall, leading to the accumulation of water and electrolytes in the gut lumen. The second mechanism is increased production of fluid in the intestine through the action of the laxative on cyclic adenosine monophosphate (cAMP) and prostaglandins, which promote active secretory processes in the intestinal mucosa.

It is also thought that stimulant laxatives may cause direct damage to mucosal cells, thereby increasing the permeability of these cells and allowing fluid to leak out.

The time taken for individual stimulant laxatives to have an effect varies according to their site of action, which may be the small intestine, the large intestine or both, but they normally work within 4–12 hours of administration. For this reason, doses are usually taken at bedtime to produce an effect the next morning. Suppository presentations (e.g. bisacodyl) produce much faster results, usually within an hour.

Cautions and contraindications

The main adverse effects of stimulant laxatives are griping and intestinal cramps. Prolonged use can result in fluid and electrolyte imbalance, and loss of colonic smooth muscle tone. This can lead to a vicious circle in which larger and larger doses of laxative are needed to produce evacuation, until eventually the bowel ceases to respond at all and constipation becomes permanent.

Stimulant laxatives should only be used for short periods – a few days at most – to re-establish bowel habit. They are not contraindicated in pregnancy but should be avoided in the first trimester, and in the last few weeks, as they may stimulate uterine contractions.

Stimulant laxatives are generally not recommended, and most are not licensed, for use in children under 5 years of age.

Certain cautions should be observed in the use of anthraquinones (see below) in view of their side-effects. They are secreted in breast milk and large doses may cause increased gastric motility and diarrhoea in infants; this class of laxative should therefore be avoided by breastfeeding mothers.

Anthraquinone glycosides are excreted via the kidney and may colour the urine a yellowish-brown to red colour depending on its pH.

Subclasses of stimulant laxatives

Several stimulant laxative agents are contained in products marketed for over-the-counter sale. They fall into two main groups: diphenylmethane derivatives and anthraquinones.

Diphenylmethane derivatives

Compounds available are:

- bisacodyl
- sodium picosulfate

Bisacodyl acts mainly via stimulation of the mucosal nerve plexus of the large intestine and so takes rather longer to act (6–10 hours) than laxatives that act within the small intestine. It is minimally absorbed and appears to exert no systemic effects. Bisacodyl causes gastric irritation; there are therefore no oral liquid presentations, and tablets are enteric coated. Tablets should be swallowed whole and should not be taken within 1 hour of an antacid. as this will lead to dissolution of the coating and release of the drug into the stomach.

Sodium picosulfate becomes active following metabolism by colonic bacteria; it therefore has a relatively slow onset of action, usually acting within 10–14 hours. It is useful in young children.

Dosages of these preparations are as follows.

- **Bisacodyl:** by mouth – adults and children over 10 years of age, 5–10 mg at night; by rectum – adults and children over 10 years of age, 10 mg (one suppository), children under 10 years of age (under medical supervision only), 5 mg (one paediatric suppository). Suppositories should be administered in the morning as they act within 15–60 minutes. Bisacodyl suppositories may cause a burning sensation in the rectum.

- **Sodium picosulfate:** adults and children over 10 years of age, 5–15 mg at night; children aged 2–10 years, 2.5–5 mg, according to age.

The following products are available.

- Bisacodyl
    - Bisacodyl tablets (5 mg; non-proprietary)
    - Biolax tablets
      Chatfield Laboratories
    - Dulco-lax tablets and Dulco-lax adults' and children's suppositories
      Boehringer Ingelheim

- Sodium picosulfate
    - Dulco-lax Perles
    - Laxoberal elixir
      both *Boehringer Ingelheim*

Anthraquinones

Anthraquinones are naturally occurring glycosides, used in the form of standardised plant extracts. They are hydrolysed by colonic bacteria to release derivatives of 1,8-dihydroxyanthraquinone, which are absorbed to a moderate degree but with little systemic consequence.

They are believed to act through a combination of direct stimulation of the intramural nerve plexus and interference with absorption of water across the intestinal wall. The effects of individual preparations vary according to the speed of hydrolysis of the glycosides they contain and their anthraquinone constituents. Preparations derived from several plant sources were popular ingredients of laxative products for many years, but in recent years have mainly dropped out of use. With the exception of senna, they are now only found in herbal laxative medicines, which generally contain mixtures of plant-derived materials rather than a single constituent.

Senna

Senna is obtained from the dried leaves or pods of *Cassia senna* (= *C. acutifolia*) (known as Alexandrian senna) or *C. angustifolia* (Tinnevelly senna). Preparations are usually standardised to the content of sennoside B (7.5 mg per tablet or 5 mL syrup).

Dosages of senna are: adults, 15 mg at night; children aged 6–12 years, 7.5 mg. (Califig, which contains senna in fig syrup, is licensed for use in children from 1 year at a dose from 1.25 mg.)

Senna is available in the following products:

- Senna Tablets 7.5 mg BP
- Califig syrup
  Merck Consumer Health

- Ex-Lax Senna chocolate
  Novartis Consumer Health

- Nylax with Senna tablets
  Crookes

- Senokot tablets, syrup and granules
- Senokot Max Strength tablets (15 mg)
  both *Reckitt Benckiser*

- Sure-Lax Senna tablets
  Chefaro UK

- Senna is also an ingredient of Manevac (Galen).

Other stimulant laxatives

Other anthraquinone plant derivatives used in over-the-counter laxative products include powdered frangula and cascara. Frangula, from the bark of *Rhamnus frangula*, is contained in Normacol Plus (Norgine) and in some herbal laxative products. Cascara, from the bark of *Rhamnus purshiana*, has a strong purgative action and griping effect. A popular laxative until a generation ago, it is now only found in herbal preparations.

Castor oil has been traditionally used as a laxative. It contains ricinoleate, which is hydrolysed in the small intestine to produce glycerol and ricinoleic acid, the latter producing a drastic purgative effect which may give rise to dehydration and electrolyte imbalance and can also cause colic. The stimulant effects are sufficient to cause uterine contraction in pregnant women and may provoke abortion. Castor oil is mentioned here because it is sometimes requested by the public as a laxative; it should not be sold for constipation under any circumstances.

Aloin is an extract of aloes obtained from the leaf gel of *Aloe barbadensis* and *A. ferox*. It has a similar but more drastic action to senna and is very irritant. Aloin is the sole constituent in Calsalettes tablets (Torbet), and aloin or powdered aloes is included in some herbal laxatives.

Osmotic laxatives

Constituents

Osmotic laxatives contain one of the following:

- magnesium sulphate
- magnesium hydroxide
- sodium sulphate
- lactulose
- macrogols (polyethylene glycols)
- glycerol.

Mode of action

Osmotic laxatives are either inorganic salts or organic compounds that are very poorly absorbed from the intestine. Their presence in the intestine creates a hypertonic state. In order to equalise osmotic pressure, water is drawn from the intestinal wall into the lumen, raising the intraluminal pressure by increasing the volume of the contents, thereby stimulating peristalsis and promoting evacuation. The effects of the inorganic salts are very rapid: large doses produce a semifluid or watery evacuation within 3 hours and smaller doses act in 6–8 hours. Magnesium salts are also believed to act by stimulating secretion of the hormone cholecystokinin, which promotes fluid secretion and motility in the intestine.

Lactulose, a synthetic disaccharide, takes much longer to act than the inorganic osmotic laxatives because it has first to be broken down by colonic bacteria, mainly to lactic acid. This produces a local osmotic effect. It may take 72 hours of regular dosing to produce an effect, which is seen as a disadvantage by patients seeking rapid results. It has a sweet taste which makes it more palatable for children, to whom it can be given safely, but many adults find the large dose volumes required (up to 30 mL) sickly and a deterrent to compliance.

Macrogols are condensation polymers of ethylene oxide and water. Two macrogols (with molecular weights of approximately 3350 and 4000) are used as osmotic laxatives. They appear to act more effectively and rapidly than lactulose, and have been suggested as the laxative of first choice for constipation in children.[5,6] Macrogols are presented as powders to be dissolved in water and are taken as a single daily dose.

Glycerol is a highly hygroscopic trihydric alcohol which appears to exert its principal laxative action by attracting water of hydration into the intestine. It is also believed to have a direct mild irritant effect and may also have some lubricating and softening actions. Glycerol is administered in the form of suppositories, which usually act within 15–30 minutes. It is a useful treatment for babies and young children. Glycerol is inactive by mouth, as it is readily absorbed and extensively metabolised in the liver.

Sorbitol is a polyhydric alcohol with a similar action to glycerol. It is not used as a laxative but is commonly employed as a sweetener in sugar-free confectionery and medicines. Unlike glycerol, it is poorly absorbed from the gastrointestinal tract; regular consumption of products containing sorbitol can cause diarrhoea.

Cautions and side-effects

Some absorption of inorganic laxative salt ions does occur, but, in normal, healthy individuals, the amounts are too small to cause toxic effects and the ions are rapidly excreted via the kidney. However, accumulation of magnesium ions can occur in the presence of renal impairment, causing toxic effects in the central nervous system and altered neuromuscular function through hypermagnesaemia. As renal function tends to decline with age, it may be advisable to discourage regular use of magnesium-containing laxatives by elderly patients.

Absorption of sodium salts can result in water retention and a rise in blood pressure; regular use should be avoided in patients with renal insufficiency, oedema, high blood pressure or congestive heart failure.

The main side-effects of inorganic osmotic laxatives are nausea and vomiting. In addition, large doses can produce significant dehydration, so sufficient water should always be drunk with a dose to ensure that there is no net loss of body water. Serious adverse effects with lactulose are rare. Relatively minor side-effects, although they may be sufficient to discourage compliance, occur in about 20% of patients taking full doses and include flatulence, cramp and abdominal discomfort, particularly at the start of treatment. Lactulose is a disaccharide of galactose and fructose and also includes some lactose. It is therefore not suitable for patients with galactose or lactose intolerance and must be used with caution in patients with diabetes.

Products

- Magnesium sulphate
  - Epsom Salts
  - Andrews Original Salts
    GSK Consumer Healthcare

- Magnesium hydroxide
  - Magnesium Hydroxide Mixture BP (Cream of Magnesia)
  - Milk of Magnesia liquid
    GSK Consumer Healthcare
  - Milpar (also contains liquid paraffin)
    Merck Consumer Health

- Sodium sulphate
  - Glauber's Salt

- Lactulose
  - Duphalac solution
    Solvay
  - Lactugal solution
    Intrapharm
  - Regulose solution
    Novartis Consumer Healthcare

- Glycerol
  - Glycerol Suppositories BP (70% in a gelatin base – mould sizes: 4 g for adults, 2 g for children, 1 g for infants)
  - Senokot Direct Relief suppositories
    Reckitt Benckiser

- Macrogols
  - Idrolax (macrogol '4000')
    Schwarz
  - Movicol, Movicol-Half and Movicol Paediatric Plain
    (macrogol 3350)
    Norgine

Faecal softener – docusate sodium

This is the only compound available.

Mode of action and cautions

Docusate sodium (dioctyl sodium sulphosuccinate) is an anionic surfactant which acts by lowering the surface tension of the intestinal contents. This allows fluid and fat to penetrate, emulsify and soften faecal material for easier elimination. The faeces are kept soft and evacuation is achieved without straining. Docusate is also thought to exert a stimulant laxative effect similar to that of the anthraquinones. A laxative effect usually occurs within 1–3 days of administration.

Used alone, docusate is a weak laxative; however, it is considered useful for patients in whom straining at stool must be avoided, for example, following an operation or myocardial infarction.

Docusate is non-absorbable and non-toxic, but it is believed to facilitate the transport of other drugs across the intestine and could thereby increase their action and adverse effects.

Dose

Adults, up to 500 mg daily in divided doses; children, 12.5–25 mg three times a day; infants over 6 months of age, 12.5 mg three times a day.

Products

- Dioctyl capsules (100 mg)
  Schwarz

- Docusol Adult solution (50 mg/5 mL) and Paediatric solution
  (12.5 mg/5 mL)
  Typharm

Faecal lubricant – liquid paraffin

Liquid paraffin is the only compound available.

Mode of action and side-effects

Liquid paraffin is indigestible and absorbed to only a small extent. It penetrates and softens the faeces and coats the surface with an oily film, facilitating passage of the faeces through the intestine.

Liquid paraffin is considered to have a limited usefulness as an occasional laxative in situations where straining at stool must be avoided, but it has several drawbacks that make it unsuitable for regular use: it can seep from the anus and cause irritation; it may interfere with the absorption of fat-soluble vitamins; it is slightly absorbed into the intestinal wall, where it may set up foreign-body granulomatous reactions; it may enter the lung through aspiration and cause lipoid pneumonia.

It should not be used in the presence of abdominal pain, nausea or vomiting and should never be used for children.

Products

The only product available is Liquid Paraffin Oral Emulsion BP (nonproprietary), but liquid paraffin is an ingredient of Milpar (Merck Consumer Health).

PRODUCT SELECTION POINTS

- Ideally, simple or functional constipation should be corrected by increasing fibre and fluid intake. These measures are not always successful, but should be tried first.
- Bulk-forming laxatives are the first-choice for the treatment of constipation. They are not absorbed, are pharmacologically inert and exert their effect by mimicking the natural action of food on the gut. They can be used long term if necessary.
- The short-term use of stimulant laxatives is justified to re-establish a bowel habit if dietary measures and bulk-forming laxatives have failed. Bisacodyl or a standardised senna preparation are the best choices. They are reliable, act relatively quickly and generally produce few side-effects. There is little to commend the use of other laxatives in this class.
- Regular use of inorganic osmotic laxatives should be avoided in the elderly and by patients with cardiovascular problems or renal impairment.
- Several factors may deter patients from using lactulose: it must be taken for up to 3 days to produce an effect, it is intensely sweet, it may cause cramping and flatulence, and it is relatively expensive. Macrogol may be a better choice of osmotic laxative.
- There is no justification for the use of liquid paraffin as a non-prescription laxative.
- Constipation is common in the later stages of pregnancy. Bulk-forming laxatives and lactulose are suitable and safe to use, although the former may add to abdominal discomfort. Breast-feeding mothers should avoid senna.
- Medical opinion is that the use of laxatives in children is undesirable and, if necessary, should only be under medical supervision. However, if dietary means fail, a single glycerol suppository of the appropriate size may be sufficient to correct the problem. Several other products are licensed for use in children, and have recommended doses.
- Constipation is often a side-effect of prescribed medication. Before recommending a laxative, the pharmacist should consult

with the patient's doctor to see if an alternative drug can be prescribed.

- Pharmacists should be alert to laxative abuse, both intentional and unwitting.

PRODUCT RECOMMENDATIONS

- First-line – dietary (i.e. increased fibre and fluid intake).
- Second-line – bulk-forming laxatives.
- Third-line – a short course of a stimulant laxative, either bisacodyl or standardised senna.
- Refer the patient if constipation is not resolved within a week.

REFERENCES

1. Ramkumar D, Rao SS. Efficacy and safety of traditional medical therapies for chronic constipation: systematic review. *Am J Gastroenterol* 2005; 100: 936–971.
2. Jones MP, Talley NJ, Nuyts G, Dubois D. Lack of objective evidence of efficacy of laxatives in chronic constipation. *Dig Dis Sci* 2002; 47: 2222–2230.
3. Petticrew M, Rodgers M, Booth A. Effectiveness of laxatives in adults. *Qual Health Care* 2001; 10: 268–273.
4. Tramonte SM, Brand MB, Mulrow CD, *et al.* The treatment of chronic constipation in adults. A systematic review. *J Gen Intern Med* 1997; 12: 15–24.
5. Fritz E, Hammer HF, Lipp RW, *et al.* Effects of lactulose and polyethylene glycol on colonic transit. *Aliment Pharmacol Ther* 2005; 21: 259–268.
6. Voskuijl W, de Lorijn F, Verwijs W, *et al.* PEG 3350 (Transipeg) versus lactulose in the treatment of childhood functional constipation: a double blind, randomised, controlled, multicentre trial. *Gut* 2004; 53: 1590–1594.

Corns and calluses

Corns and calluses are localised formations of thick, horny skin (hyperkeratinisation) on the feet.

CAUSES

Corns and calluses are caused by pressure or friction on the feet. Pressure on the nerve endings in these areas gives rise to pain. Hard corns occur over bony prominences, generally on or around the toes; soft corns occur between the toes and have a soft and whitened appearance caused by maceration of the skin by perspiration. Calluses form on the flatter, weight-bearing and fleshier areas of the foot.

TREATMENT

Treatment is by epidermabrasion or the use of hydrocolloid plasters or keratolytic agents.

Cautions with 'at-risk' patients

Particular care is needed with certain groups of at-risk patients. Patients with diabetes, for example, often have poor peripheral circulation; they are therefore more liable to ischaemic foot lesions than healthy people, and will recover less readily from any minor foot damage. In addition, peripheral neuropathy may result in a decreased perception of pain so that any injury to the feet may not be noticed. Vision may also be impaired, particularly in elderly patients with diabetes, making it more difficult to see any damage that may have occurred. Pharmacists should not, therefore, recommend any treatment for foot problems to patients with diabetes and, if asked for advice, should refer the patient to either a chiropodist or their doctor. This caution also applies to patients with peripheral vascular disease and to the elderly who, like patients with diabetes, tend to have more foot problems, may have declining peripheral circulatory and sensory nerve function, and often do not have the physical mobility or the dexterity to manage their own treatment properly.

Epidermabrasion

Epidermabrasion does not involve the use of pharmacological agents but is a physical process that involves removal of the horny skin by the use of a mechanical aid. Several gently abrasive materials and appliances are available, ranging from emery boards and pumice stones to specially designed files such as the Scholl corn and callus file (SSL International), and synthetic pumice-like blocks such as Newton's Foot Therapy chiropody sponge (Brodie & Stone).

Careful technique is important for the successful and safe removal of hard skin by epidermabrasion, and the following are the main points of advice that should be given to patients.

- Soak the foot (to soften the skin) in mild soapy water for a few minutes, or apply a moisturising or softening cream.
- Rub some soap onto the appliance, and gently rub the corn or callus for 5 minutes.
- Repeat the process nightly for 1 week, then review. There is no need to remove the hard skin completely, just enough to relieve pain or irritation.
- Do not wear ill-fitting shoes (often the cause of the hyperkeratinisation), to help prevent recurrence of the problem.

Hydrocolloid and hydrogel plasters

Hydrocolloids and hydrogels are complex polymer formulations used in wound management. They swell in the presence of moisture absorbed from the skin; in corn and callus plasters, the hydrocolloid or hydrogel forms a soft, protective gel-like cushion which rehydrates and softens the hardened tissue. The plaster is left *in situ* for about a week; the corn or callused skin should be removed when the plaster is removed.

Examples of products:

- Compeed Hydrocure system for calluses and corns
  J&J

- Scholl Corn Clear Gel Plasters
  SSL International

Keratolytic agent – salicylic acid

Mode of action and use

In the removal of corns and calluses, the function of salicylic acid is to remove a thick layer of cornified skin cells, mainly through loosening the attachment of the area of hardened skin to the normal skin (see chapter on Athlete's foot).

The concentration of salicylic acid in products used for this purpose ranges from about 11 to 50%, depending on the type of formulation.

Corn and callus caps and plasters contain high concentrations of salicylic acid (usually 40%) in a semi-solid base spread onto a suitable backing material, contained within a ring that is either self-adhesive or attached to an adhesive plaster. Such systems provide direct and prolonged contact with the affected area. They should be applied and changed every 1 or 2 days for about a week, after which time the callosity should lift away easily. If the callosity cannot be removed after 10–14 days' treatment, professional help should be sought. An ointment containing 50% salicylic acid is also available; it should be applied nightly for 4 nights.

Paints and liquids that contain salicylic acid in a concentration of 11–17% are available, often in a collodion-based vehicle. Collodions contain pyroxylin, a nitrocellulose derivative, dissolved in a volatile solvent such as ether, acetone or alcohol. On application, the solvent evaporates, leaving on the skin an adherent, flexible, water-repellent film containing the medicament. This has the advantage of maintaining the salicylic acid at the site of application and also assists maceration of the skin by preventing moisture evaporation. Liquid preparations are usually applied daily for several days until the corn or callus can be removed easily.

Cautions

As salicylic acid is caustic to normal skin, care should be taken to prevent preparations from spreading beyond affected areas. True sensitivity to salicylic acid is very rare, but a few patients react to colophony present in collodions and plaster bases. Preparations containing high concentrations of salicylic acid should be avoided by patients who are sensitive to aspirin.

Product examples

- Carnation Corn Caps
- Carnation Callus Caps
  both *Cuxson Gerrard*

- Scholl Corn Removal Plasters (washproof)
- Scholl Callus Removal Pads
  both *SSL International*

- Pickles Foot Ointment
  Ransom

- Salicylic Acid Collodion BP

- Dispello Corn & Wart Paint
  Ayrton Saunders

- Bazuka (Dendron) and Salatac (Dermal) (both contain 4% lactic acid in combination with 12% salicylic acid and are licensed for the treatment of corns and calluses; see also chapters on Verrucas and Warts).

PRODUCT SELECTION POINTS

- Epidermabrasion or hydrocolloid plasters are the safest and most suitable methods for treating corns and calluses.

- A wide range of preparations containing salicylic acid is available, all of which should be effective if properly used.

PRODUCT RECOMMENDATIONS

- First-line treatment – epidermabrasion or hydrocolloid plasters.
- Second-line treatment – plasters or a liquid application containing salicylic acid.

Cough

(continued . . .)

Cough associated with an upper respiratory tract infection is generally treated with medicines that are available without prescription, but there is disagreement about their effectiveness. The conclusion of a Cochrane systematic review was that: 'over the counter cough medicines for acute cough cannot be recommended because there is no good evidence for their effectiveness'.[1] On the other hand, there can be little doubt of the faith that the general public has in non-prescription cough treatments, with a total of more than 80 proprietary brands and variants on the market and sales in excess of £100 million in the UK in 2004. However, there is no good evidence for or against the effectiveness of over-the-counter (OTC) medicines in acute cough, partly because there is a lack of sufficiently large and well-designed clinical trials on which to base a confident conclusion.[1] Trials of individual constituents have produced conflicting results, but most have not been shown to be entirely ineffective. As in many areas of self-medication, placebo effect must be expected to play a significant part in perception of the effectiveness of cough remedies; however, it has been proposed that cough syrups may have a pharmacological action, as a sweet taste may modulate cough at the level of the nucleus tractus solitarius in the brain, possibly by influencing the production of endogenous opioids.[2]

NATURE OF COUGHS

There are three types of cough:

- dry (irritating and non-productive)
- chesty with production of mucus
- chesty but non-productive (no mucus is produced but there is a feeling of 'tightness' or wheezing resulting from congestion of the bronchial airways).

Product choice depends on the type of cough. The active ingredients of cough remedies fall into four main categories:

- suppressants, to treat dry, irritating coughs
- expectorants for chesty, productive coughs
- decongestants for chesty, non-productive coughs
- demulcents, to soothe any kind of cough.

Products that contain combinations of ingredients should be selected carefully to ensure that they are suitable for the symptoms and that the combination is rational.

TREATMENT OF DRY IRRITATING COUGHS – SUPPRESSANTS (ANTITUSSIVES)

Two classes of compounds – opioids and antihistamines – are used as antitussives in cough preparations.

Opioids

Compounds available

Compounds available are:

- codeine
- pholcodine
- dextromethorphan.

Mode of action

Infection of the upper respiratory tract produces inflammation and irritation of the throat and trachea, stimulating the cough reflex in an attempt to remove what the brain perceives as a foreign object, resulting in a dry, non-productive cough. Such coughing serves no beneficial purpose, is inconvenient and can eventually become debilitating. It can justifiably be suppressed with antitussives.

Opium alkaloids act on the medullary cough centre in the brain to depress the cough reflex. Both dextro and laevo isomers of opioid compounds possess antitussive activity, but only the laevo isomers have liability for dependence.

Dextromethorphan, a dextro isomer developed as an orally active antitussive with little or no dependence liability, is now the most widely used opioid constituent of OTC cough remedies.

Recent evidence as to whether codeine, pholcodine and dextromethorphan are effective is conflicting, and most trials rate them as little or no better than placebo.[3–7] Codeine and pholcodine have been traditionally rated as more potent than dextromethorphan.

Dosage

- **Codeine:** adults, 15–30 mg three or four times daily; children aged 5–12 years, half adult dose; children aged 1–5 years, 3 mg three or four times daily (not suitable for infants under 1 year)
- **Pholcodine:** adults, 5–10 mg three or four times daily; children aged 1–12 years, 2.5–5 mg three or four times daily; infants aged 3–12 months, 1 mg three or four times daily; pharmacokinetic studies have shown pholcodine to have a long half-life, and twice-, or even once-, daily dosing may be sufficient.
- **Dextromethorphan:** adults, 10–20 mg every 4 hours; children aged 6–12 years, 5–15 mg up to 4 hourly to a maximum of 60 mg in 24 hours; children aged 1–6 years, 2.5–5 mg to a maximum of 30 mg in 24 hours.

Cautions and side-effects

Codeine is partially demethylated in the body to morphine. This may contribute to its antitussive activity but also accounts for its liability to cause sedation, respiratory depression (although this is not normally a problem at OTC doses), constipation and addiction.

Codeine is now little used in proprietary formulations. Pholcodine has a generally better side-effect profile than codeine, and dextromethorphan is claimed to be virtually free from side-effects.

Interactions

At antitussive doses, opioids have no significant interactions with other drugs.

Product examples

- Codeine
  — Codeine Linctus BP (no proprietary product marketed primarily for OTC sale contains codeine as sole constituent)

- Pholcodine
  — Pholcodine Linctus BP

  — Galenphol Linctus
    Thornton & Ross

  — Tixylix daytime
    Novartis Consumer Health

- Dextromethorphan
  — Robitussin Dry Coughs
    Wyeth

Many products contain opioids in combination with other ingredients. The use of combination cough remedies is discussed below.

Antihistamines

Compounds available

Compounds available are:

- brompheniramine
- diphenhydramine
- promethazine
- triprolidine.

Mode of action and efficacy

The above compounds are all sedating-type antihistamines and exert a central and peripheral inhibitory action on neuronal pathways involved in the cough reflex. The sedative properties of these compounds may be an important factor in their use, insofar as they will help cough sufferers to sleep if taken near bedtime. They also exert anticholinergic side-effects, including the drying up of bronchial and nasal secretions, which may be helpful in some situations.

Little research has been published on the antitussive effects of antihistamines, but trials that have been performed show that they are effective.[8,9]

Uses

As for opioids.

Dosage

The maximum dose recommended by the manufacturers of cough remedies containing diphenhydramine and triprolidine is at the lower end of the therapeutic range for these compounds. The two products containing promethazine contain quantities that appear to be below the therapeutic level.

Side-effects and cautions

Side-effects include sedation, and anticholinergic effects such as dry mouth, urinary retention, constipation and blurring of vision. The elderly are more susceptible to these side-effects. Because of these side-effects, cough preparations containing antihistamines should not be recommended to patients with glaucoma or prostate problems. Paradoxical stimulation of the central nervous system (CNS) can also occur, particularly in children, and there have been occasional reports of hallucinatory episodes.

Interactions

The sedative effects of antidepressants, anxiolytics and hypnotics are likely to be enhanced by antihistamines, as are the antimuscarinic actions and side-effects of drugs such as trihexyphenidyl, orphenadrine, tricyclic antidepressants and phenothiazines.

Product examples

- Brompheniramine: Dimotane range
  Wyeth

- Diphenhydramine: some products in the Benylin range
  Pfizer Consumer Healthcare

- Promethazine: Tixylix Night-Time SF
  Novartis Consumer Health

- Triprolidine: Actifed Dry Cough and Actifed Chesty Cough
  Pfizer Consumer Healthcare

TREATMENT OF CHESTY, PRODUCTIVE COUGHS – EXPECTORANTS

Compounds available

Compounds available are:

- guaifenesin
- ammonium chloride
- ipecacuanha
- squill.

Mode of action and efficacy

In a productive cough, mucus produced in the bronchial passages as a result of infection is moved upwards towards the pharynx by ciliary action and is then expelled by coughing. As the cough is clearing mucus and helping to keep the airways open, it should not be suppressed.

Expectorants are used to assist mucus removal. In large doses they are emetic, however, acting through vagal stimulation of the gastric mucosa to produce a reflex response from the vomiting centre in the brain. The same mechanism stimulates the bronchial glands and cilia and it is postulated that this stimulation still occurs at sub-emetic doses.

Although expectorants have long been used in the treatment of cough, there is little objective evidence of their effectiveness. Guaifenesin is frequently used in proprietary preparations, and is recognised by the US Food and Drug Administration as being effective at doses of around 200 mg three times a day. However, the drug has a short half-life and more frequent dosing may be necessary to ensure effectiveness.

As is often the case with OTC products, many expectorant preparations contain what appear to be sub-therapeutic levels of constituents. Manufacturers may do this to reduce to an absolute minimum the possibility of any adverse effects from substances for which, even at full doses, there is little proof of efficacy. Even at the highest strengths included in OTC formulations there is little risk of adverse effects, and expectorants do not interact with other drugs.

Product examples

The following products contain guaifenesin as the sole constituent.

- Hill's Balsam Chesty Cough Liquid
  LPC

- Robitussin Chesty Coughs
  Wyeth

- Jackson's All Fours
  Herbal Concepts

- Tixylix Chesty Cough
  Novartis Consumer Health

TREATMENT OF CHESTY, NON-PRODUCTIVE COUGHS – DECONGESTANTS

Compounds from two groups are used as decongestants and bronchodilators in cough remedies: sympathomimetics and a methylxanthine (theophylline).

Sympathomimetics

Compounds available

Compounds available are:

- ephedrine
- pseudoephedrine.

Action, uses and dosage

Sympathomimetics mimic the action of noradrenaline (norepinephrine), the principal neurotransmitter between the nerve endings of the sympathetic nervous system and the adrenergic receptors of the innervated tissues. They stimulate both alpha adrenoceptors, causing constriction of smooth muscle and blood vessels, and beta adrenoceptors, producing bronchodilatation. They are therefore useful in coughs where the tissues of the upper respiratory tract are congested, as they shrink swollen mucosae and open up the airways. Sympathomimetics may also have CNS-stimulating effects and their vasoconstricting action tends to raise blood pressure.

The two sympathomimetics used in cough preparations have more or less equivalent action on the respiratory tract, but ephedrine has greater CNS and pressor activity and is used in few products. The recommended adult doses of pseudoephedrine is 60 mg up to four times daily, and for ephedrine is up to 60 mg three times a day.

Side-effects and cautions

Because of their pressor effects, and because they can also increase heart rate, sympathomimetic decongestants should be avoided by patients with any kind of cardiovascular condition or glaucoma. These drugs also interfere with metabolism, including glucose metabolism, and should not be taken by patients with diabetes or thyroid problems. As they are CNS stimulants, doses should not be taken near to bedtime.

Interactions

Monoamine oxidase inhibitors (MAOIs) prevent the breakdown of noradrenaline and increase the amount stored in adrenergic nerve terminals. Administration of sympathomimetics in conjunction with MAOIs will increase the level of adrenergic transmitter substances, potentially resulting in a lethal hypertensive crisis. Sympathomimetic decongestants must therefore not be given to patients taking MAOIs.

Oral decongestants should also be avoided by patients taking beta-blockers. Sympathomimetics stimulate both the alpha adrenoceptors of the cardiovascular system to produce vasoconstriction, and the beta adrenoceptors to produce vasodilatation and stimulation of the heart. The overall effect is a slight increase in both blood pressure and heart rate. Blockade of beta-adrenoceptors by beta-blockers allows unopposed alpha-adrenoceptor-mediated vasoconstriction, which can lead to a greater and potentially hazardous rise in blood pressure.

Product examples

- Pseudoephedrine (in combination products)
  - Actifed Multi Action Chesty
    Pfizer Consumer Healthcare
  - Dimotane Expectorant
    Wyeth
  - Meltus Adult Expectorant with Decongestant
    SSL International

- Ephedrine
  - Do-Do Chesteze Tablets
    Novartis Consumer Health

Theophylline

Action, uses and dosage

Bronchodilatation is mediated by cyclic adenosine monophosphate (cAMP), which causes smooth muscle relaxation through intracellular modulation of calcium ion levels. cAMP is depleted when bronchoconstriction occurs, being broken down by the enzyme phosphodiesterase (PDE). Theophylline is thought to preferentially inhibit PDE type IV, which is found in smooth bronchial muscle.

Theophylline is used mainly in the treatment of asthma, but it is included in one OTC product – Do-Do Chesteze tablets (Novartis Consumer Health) – marketed for the treatment of bronchial cough, breathlessness and wheezing.

Interactions and cautions

Theophylline is metabolised in the liver and interacts with several commonly prescribed drugs that inhibit its metabolism, causing serum levels to rise. This is important because theophylline has a narrow therapeutic index, and concentrations can rise rapidly to toxic levels. Commonly used drugs that show significant interactions with theophylline include: cimetidine, ciprofloxacin (and other quinolone antibacterials), erythromycin (and other macrolides), fluvoxamine, St John's wort, calcium-channel blockers and fluconazole. Smoking speeds up the metabolism of theophylline, necessitating larger doses.

Theophylline should be used with caution in patients with liver or cardiac disease, epilepsy, the elderly, and pregnant and breastfeeding women.

In view of the problems associated with theophylline, and the availability of a wide range of alternative treatments, it would seem best not to recommend any theophylline-containing OTC product (only one product is available).

TREATMENT TO SOOTHE ANY KIND OF COUGH – DEMULCENTS

Compounds available are:

- glycerol
- liquid glucose
- syrup
- honey
- treacle.

Action and uses

Demulcents coat the mucosa of the pharynx and provide short-lived relief of the irritation that provokes reflex coughing. They are used mainly for their placebo effect, although a possible true pharmacological effect has been proposed.[2] Pastilles (e.g. glycerin (glycerol), lemon and honey) provide a more prolonged soothing effect as they promote production of saliva, which has a demulcent effect while the pastille is being sucked. Demulcents can be safely taken by anyone, the only drawback being the high sugar content of some preparations, so these should be used with caution in patients with diabetes and in children because of their cariogenic potential. Several sugar-free linctuses are available, both of the demulcent type and containing active ingredients.

Product examples

- Glycerin, Lemon and Honey Linctus (non-proprietary)
- Simple Linctus BP
- Meltus Baby Cough Linctus
  SSL International

TREATMENT WITH COMBINATION REMEDIES

Proprietary cough remedies that contain a single ingredient are the exception rather than the rule. Some products contain just an antitussive (usually dextromethorphan) or an expectorant (usually guaifenesin), but the majority are mixtures containing up to six ingredients, plus vehicle and flavourings. Many products contain pharmacologically rational combinations, such as an antitussive with a decongestant/bronchodilator, which is sensible for a dry cough with wheeziness or congestion, or an expectorant with a decongestant, suitable for a productive cough with congestion.

The number of irrational formulations has been reduced in recent years, but there are still some available that combine an expectorant with an antihistamine, which have mutually antagonistic effects on clearance of mucus, or that combine an antitussive to suppress coughing with an expectorant to promote it.

Some products contain, in addition to a more or less therapeutic quantity of an active constituent, a number of 'traditional' ingredients in very small concentrations. It is unlikely that these could have any therapeutic effect, and they are presumably included to present a suitably impressive formula on the label to increase placebo effect. Menthol and volatile oils, which provide a suitably 'medicinal' aroma and flavour, are also often included.

Some products contain sub-therapeutic amounts of several ingredients with the same action, such as expectorants, perhaps in the belief that they will have an additive effect and be effective while minimising any adverse effects. Such combinations are unlikely to have any therapeutic effect beyond that of a placebo.

PRODUCT SELECTION POINTS

- The symptoms and history of a cough should be assessed carefully and diagnosed as trivial before recommending any OTC treatment. Coughs that persist for more than 2 weeks should be referred for further investigation.
- Placebo effect may play a more important part in the perceived effectiveness of cough remedies than in most other groups of OTC products. Nevertheless, many products do contain constituents with at least a degree of recognised effectiveness. Products should be chosen rationally, with ingredients matched to symptoms, and the possibility of contraindications and interactions taken into account.
- Cough suppressants are indicated for dry, irritating, non-productive coughs; expectorants for productive, chesty coughs; decongestants for cough accompanied by congestion. Demulcent preparations can be used for any kind of cough, are harmless and have a useful placebo effect.
- Combinations of a suppressant or an expectorant with a decongestant are appropriate for certain types of cough. Other combinations are irrational, and may contain antagonistic ingredients.
- Products should be selected that contain a therapeutic dose of active ingredient(s); some products contain sub-therapeutic amounts and are likely to have no effect.

- Products containing antihistamines should be used with caution in the elderly, and should be avoided in patients with glaucoma or prostatic hypertrophy.
- Products containing sympathomimetic decongestants should not be taken by patients with diabetes, glaucoma, cardiovascular or thyroid problems, or by patients taking beta-blockers or MAOIs.
- Products containing theophylline should not be taken by patients taking cimetidine, quinolone or macrolide antibacterials, fluvoxamine, St John's wort, calcium-channel blockers or fluconazole because of an interaction that can raise plasma theophylline concentrations to toxic levels.
- Sugar-free linctuses suitable for patients with diabetes and sugar-free cough medicines for children are available.

PRODUCT RECOMMENDATIONS

- Cough suppressants – pholcodine or dextromethorphan.
- Expectorants – guaifenesin, preparations containing 200 mg per adult dose.
- Non-productive cough with congestion (dry, wheezy, 'tight') – dextromethorphan with pseudoephedrine.
- Productive cough with congestion – guaifenesin with pseudoephedrine.
- Demulcents – products such Simple Linctus BP, and Glycerin, Lemon and Honey Linctus are cheap, harmless and have a useful placebo effect. They can be used for any type of cough.

REFERENCES

1. Schroeder K, Fahey T. Over-the-counter medications for acute cough in children and adults in ambulatory settings. *The Cochrane Library,* issue 4. Chichester, UK: John Wiley & Sons, 2004 (www.thecochranelibrary.com).
2. Eccles R. Mechanisms of the placebo effect of sweet cough syrups. *Respir Physiol Neurobiol* 2005; Dec 1 [Epub ahead of print].

3. Lee PCL, Jawad MS, Eccles R. Antitussive efficacy of dextromethorphan in cough associated with acute upper respiratory tract infection. *J Pharm Pharmacol* 2000; 52: 1137–1142.
4. Committee on Drugs. American Academy of Pediatrics. Use of codeine- and dextromethorphan-containing cough remedies in children. *Pediatrics* 1997; 99: 918–920.
5. Taylor JA, Novack AH, Almquist JR, Rogers JE. Efficacy of cough suppressants in children. *J Pediatr* 1993; 122: 799–802.
6. Croughan-Minihane MS, Petitti DB, Rodnick JE, Eliaser G. Clinical trial examining effectiveness of three cough syrups. *J Am Board Fam Pract* 1993; 6: 109–115.
7. Freestone C, Eccles R. Assessment of the antitussive efficacy of codeine in cough associated with common cold. *J Pharm Pharmacol* 1997; 49: 1045–1049.
8. Eccles R, Morris S, Jawad M. Lack of effect of codeine in the treatment of cough associated with acute upper respiratory tract infection. *J Clin Pharm Ther* 1992; 17: 175–180.
9. Packman EW, Ciccone PE, Wilson J, Masurat T. Antitussive effects of diphenhydramine on the citric acid aerosol-induced cough response in humans. *Int J Clin Pharmacol Ther Toxicol* 1991; 29: 218–222.
10. Curley FJ, Irwin RS, Pratter MR, *et al.* Cough and the common cold. *Am Rev Respir Dis* 1988; 138: 305–311.

Cradle cap

Cradle cap appears as scaling and crusting of the scalp in infants. Its appearance may be worrying to parents, but it is not usually serious.

CAUSES

Cradle cap is a form of seborrhoeic dermatitis of the scalp, causing scaling and crusting. It usually appears within the first 3 months of life and resolves spontaneously within a year.

TREATMENT

Products available

Four licensed products are available without prescription.

- Capasal Therapeutic Shampoo (Dermal) is a shampoo licensed for use in several scalp conditions). It contains salicylic acid, coconut oil and coal tar. It is quite expensive.
- Dentinox Cradle Cap Shampoo (Dendron) contains sodium lauryl ether sulphosuccinate and sodium lauryl ether sulphate – both anionic surfactant detergents commonly used in medicated shampoos.
- Pragmatar (Alliance) contains a cetyl alcohol-coal tar distillate with sulphur and salicylic acid. It is applied to the scalp after shampooing, and can be diluted with a little water in the palm of the hand before application. It can be used daily if necessary.
- Dandrazol Anti-Dandruff Shampoo (Transdermal) and Nizoral Dandruff Shampoo, (McNeil) are 2% ketoconazole shampoos.

Efficacy

There is no evidence that the first three treatments listed above are any more effective at treating cradle cap than the method recommended in the *British National Formulary*, which involves rubbing olive oil or arachis oil into the scalp, followed by shampooing.

Ketoconazole has been shown to be effective and safe for the treatment of infantile seborrhoeic dermatitis, but it should be reserved for serious cases and preferably used under medical supervision.[1]

REFERENCE

1.   Taieb A, Legrain V, Palmier C, *et al*. Topical ketoconazole for infantile seborrhoeic dermatitis. *Dermatologica* 1990; 181: 26–32.

Cystitis

Cystitis is inflammation of the bladder and urethra, characterised by the frequent urge to pass urine, with a burning or stinging sensation on urination.

Bacterial infection is responsible for about half of all cases, and *Escherichia coli* is the most common causative organism. *E. coli* infection results in increased acidity of the urine, which causes the inflammation that produces the symptoms of cystitis. Cystitis is relatively rare in men and is often associated with abnormalities of the genitourinary tract; men reporting symptoms of cystitis should always be referred to a doctor. Children should also be referred, as they are susceptible to permanent kidney and bladder damage as a result of urinary-tract infection (UTI).

Symptomatic treatments

Treatments that have been used traditionally for symptomatic relief are based on alkalinising agents that restore the pH of the urine to normal. However, there appears to be no clinical evidence to support their use, and one investigation found no correlation between the urine pH of women while they were suffering cystitis symptoms and after they had recovered.[1] It also found no significant differences in either symptomatology or urine pH between patients with or without significant bacteriuria. The *British National Formulary* states that alkalinising agents may relieve discomfort.

Compounds available

The alkalinising agents used are:

- sodium bicarbonate

- sodium carbonate
- sodium citrate
- potassium citrate.

Administration and dosage

Sodium bicarbonate alone is an effective alkalinising agent and is very cheap. It is kept in most homes and is useful when nothing else is to hand. The recommended dose for alkalinisation of the urine is 3 g (a level teaspoonful) in water every 2 hours until symptoms subside.

Sodium citrate is contained in several proprietary products (often together with sodium bicarbonate) for the relief of symptoms in cystitis. In each of these products the combined alkalinity of the salts is equivalent to about 4 g sodium citrate per dose.

Potassium citrate is contained in several preparations in a dose of 3 g. One product contains citric acid and potassium bicarbonate.

The recommended dosage for all these proprietary preparations is three times daily for 48 hours. The full course should be completed, even if the symptoms have gone, but patients should be referred if symptoms persist beyond the length of a course. All products should be diluted well with water, and an additional large intake of fluid is recommended to reduce the acidity of the urine through dilution and to flush any infecting organisms out of the bladder.

Cautions, contraindications and interactions

The sodium content of preparations for cystitis is high (i.e. about 35 mmol [800 mg] per dose), and can cause fluid retention and raised blood pressure. These products should therefore be avoided by patients with hypertension, heart disease, diabetes or impaired renal function and during pregnancy. (Pregnant women presenting with symptoms of cystitis should be referred to a doctor.)

Sodium-containing preparations should also be avoided by patients on lithium. Sodium is preferentially absorbed by the kidney and the excretion of lithium is increased, resulting in reduced plasma lithium concentrations.

There is a theoretical risk of hyperkalaemia if potassium citrate is taken together with potassium-sparing diuretics or other potassium-sparing drugs such as angiotensin-converting enzyme (ACE) inhibitors or aldosterone antagonists. The risk is negligible with the short courses recommended for cystitis preparations, but the advice generally given on package inserts is that patients taking any medication for cardiovascular conditions should consult their doctor.

Products

- Sodium bicarbonate
  — Sodium Bicarbonate BP
- Sodium citrate
  — Canesten Oasis sachets
    Bayer Consumer Care
  — Cymalon sachets
    Thornton & Ross
  — Cystemme sachets
    Abbott Laboratories
  — Cystocalm sachets
    Galpharm International
- Potassium citrate
  — Potassium Citrate Mixture BP
  — Cymalon cranberry liquid
    Thornton & Ross
  — Cystopurin sachets
    Bayer Consumer Care
- Citric acid and potassium citrate
  — Effercitrate effervescent tablets
    Typharm

Antibacterial treatment – trimethoprim

Mode of action and use in cystitis

Trimethoprim inhibits the enzyme dihydrofolate reductase, which facilitates the production of folic acid, itself essential to the synthesis of DNA. This biosynthetic pathway is common to humans and bacteria, but bacterial dihydrofolate reductase is many more times more sensitive to trimethoprim than the human equivalent, accounting for the drug's effectiveness and specificity. Trimethoprim is effective against a wide range of bacteria, including *E. coli*, which is responsible for 65–80% of UTIs, and other causative organisms of UTIs.

A 3-day course of trimethoprim, 200 mg twice daily, is established as an effective first-line treatment for the treatment of UTI in general practice.[2,3] It is expected that during 2006 trimethoprim will be reclassified as a Pharmacy medicine for supply to women who have had a previous diagnosis of an uncomplicated UTI. This section has been included on this expectation and progress will be reported via the 6-monthly updates on the Pharmaceutical Press website (see Preface). The rationale for reclassification to Pharmacy status includes the following points.[4]

- UTIs account for a large proportion of consultations, and uncomplicated cystitis is usually treated empirically with trimethoprim.
- Diagnosis of cystitis is nearly always made on the basis of symptoms, which is as reliable as microbial urinalysis.
- Convenience to patients can be improved and the consultation load on doctors reduced by making repeat supplies of trimethoprim available without prescription following an initial diagnosis of cystitis by a doctor.
- Resistance to trimethoprim is unlikely to be increased by making it available from pharmacies, as supplies will generally be substitutes for prescriptions. In addition, prescribing of less appropriate antibiotics may decrease. The licensing conditions (see below) are also designed to minimise the development of resistance.

- Risk of misuse is low as the drug is available only in a pack of six tablets and can be supplied only in accordance with a protocol that takes into account all the licensing conditions and restrictions.

Licensing conditions

Trimethoprim can be supplied without prescription from a pharmacy under the following conditions:

- for treatment of acute bacterial cystitis in women aged 16–70 years, who have had a diagnosis of the condition confirmed by a doctor
- a dosage of one 200 mg tablet twice daily for 3 days (i.e. the contents of a pack of six tablets)
- the treatment is contraindicated and may not be supplied, and medical referral should be made, in any of the following circumstances:
  — during pregnancy and whilst breastfeeding
  — three or more attacks of cystitis in the previous 12 months, or an attack within the previous 2 weeks
  — symptoms not improved within 72 hours of taking a course of trimethoprim
  — any untreated vaginal discharge or irritation
  — symptoms of upper UTI or pyelonephritis
  — known hypersensitivity to trimethoprim
  — known blood dyscrasias, porphyria or impaired renal function
  — trimethoprim already being taken or planned as prophylaxis of cystitis
  — known abnormality or tumour of the urinary tract
  — iatrogenic cystitis
  — males of any age.

Adverse effects and interactions

Trimethoprim has been in use for nearly 30 years and has a well-established safety and tolerability profile. The common side-effects are minor. Interactions are possible with several drugs but are generally not significant. Potentially hazardous reactions occur, and concomitant administration should be avoided, with the following: amiodarone, azathioprine, ciclosporin, mercaptopurine, methotrexate, phenytoin, procainamide, pyrimethamine.

Product

- Cysticlear
  Alpharma

PRODUCT SELECTION POINTS

- Trimethoprim is indicated for the treatment of bacterial cystitis that has been previously diagnosed by a doctor, in normal, healthy women aged 16–70 years.
- There is no clinical evidence that traditionally used alkalinising agents are effective in relieving cystitis symptoms.
- Plain sodium bicarbonate is as effective an alkalinising agent as any other treatment. Proprietary products offer the convenience of accurately measured doses and useful information on treating and coping with cystitis.
- Products containing sodium salts should not be sold to patients with hypertension or heart disease, to pregnant women or to patients taking lithium.
- The risk of hyperkalaemia from short courses of potassium-containing products is very low, but package information may deter patients who are taking medication for cardiovascular conditions from using these over-the-counter products.

PRODUCT RECOMMENDATIONS

- For women with a previous diagnosis of bacterial cystitis and no adverse indications – trimethoprim.
- For symptomatic relief – any proprietary product taking into account contraindications.

REFERENCES

1. Brumfitt W, Hamilton-Miller JM, Cooper J, Raeburn A. Relationship of urinary pH to symptoms of 'cystitis'. *Postgrad Med J* 1990; 66: 727–729.
2. Baerheim A. Empirical treatment of uncomplicated cystitis. *BMJ* 2001; 323: 1197–1198.
3. Norrby SR. Short-term treatment of uncomplicated lower urinary tract infections in women. *Rev Infect Dis* 1990; 12: 458–467.
4. MHRA. Consultation Document: ARM 30. 6 July 2005. (MHRA/PL/AL/ARM30).

Dandruff and seborrhoeic dermatitis

(continued . . .)

Dandruff is seen as excessive shedding of the cornified cells of the scalp in the form of scales. Seborrhoeic dermatitis results from accelerated epidermal proliferation and sebaceous gland activity on the scalp, face and trunk.

Dandruff

Dandruff (pityriasis capitis) is a chronic, non-inflammatory scalp condition characterised by excessive shedding of the cornified cells of the scalp in the form of scales, which is sometimes accompanied by itching and redness of the scalp. Dandruff is rare in young children, but incidence increases rapidly with age, peaking in the second decade of life and declining gradually thereafter. Estimates of prevalence vary, but it has been claimed that 75% of the population is affected by dandruff at some time in their lives. It appears to affect both sexes equally.

Dandruff is caused by increases in the production of horny substance and cell turnover on the scalp, and may be associated with raised androgen levels. It has been claimed that the condition is a normal physiological state that has become elevated to the status of a disease solely on cosmetic grounds. However, people with dandruff have been found to have high levels of microorganisms on the scalp, particularly the yeast *Pityrosporum ovale*, compared with those who do not have the condition. It has not been determined conclusively whether this organism is the cause of dandruff or is merely encouraged by the abundance of nutrients from shed skin cells; however, antimicrobial shampoos active against *P. ovale* appear to control the condition.

Seborrhoeic dermatitis

Seborrhoeic dermatitis (seborrhoea) is the result of accelerated epidermal proliferation and sebaceous gland activity on the scalp, face and trunk. On the scalp, the condition may be difficult to distinguish from more severe forms of dandruff, as characteristic features are the presence of greasy scales and often pruritus. Seborrhoeic dermatitis is common in infants, when it is known as cradle cap (see chapter on Cradle cap), relatively rare in children and occurs again from puberty, the incidence peaking between the ages of 18 and 40 years.

The condition may also involve the area in and around the ears, the eyebrows and eyelashes. As in dandruff, growth of *P. ovale* is increased in the scaly epidermis and may be a causative agent – a theory supported by the fact that ketoconazole improves the condition.

TREATMENT

Topical treatments for dandruff and mild forms of seborrhoeic dermatitis are the same and are available without prescription. Regular use (at least twice weekly) of an ordinary mild detergent shampoo will effectively control dandruff by removing scales.

A wide range of medicated treatments is available, containing ingredients such as:

- pyrithione zinc
- selenium sulphide
- ketoconazole
- coal tar
- keratolytic agents
- antimicrobial detergents.

Pyrithione zinc and selenium sulphide

Mode of action

Both compounds are cytostatic agents, which act by reducing the rate of epidermal cell turnover. The compounds are generally accepted as being effective in controlling dandruff and are of approximately equal efficacy.[1] The action of pyrithione zinc is thought to involve a non-specific toxicity for epidermal cells, whereas selenium sulphide is believed to have a direct antimitotic effect. It has also been suggested that selenium sulphide has an inhibitory action against *P. ovale*, exerted by irreversibly changing free sulphydryl groups in the yeast cells into rigid polysulphide bonds, thereby preventing cell division.

Administration

The effectiveness of pyrithione zinc depends on the extent of binding to the hair and epidermis, which is a function of time, temperature, concentration and frequency of application. Early formulations required contact times of 5–10 minutes, but for current products 2–3 minutes twice or three times weekly is sufficient.

Selenium sulphide is used twice weekly for 2 weeks, then weekly as necessary to control the condition. Each of the two applications per treatment should be left on the hair for 3 minutes.

Contraindications, cautions and side-effects

Pyrithione zinc binds strongly to both the hair and epidermis but does not penetrate into the dermis; long-term use has not been associated with toxicity. Selenium sulphide also appears safe for long-term external use, although it is highly toxic if ingested. Regular use of selenium sulphide shampoo tends to leave a residual odour of hydrogen sulphide and makes the scalp oily. Hair should not be dyed or permed for at least 2 days before or after using the shampoo. Contact dermatitis and hypersensitivity are possible but rare with both compounds. Neither compound should be applied to broken or abraded skin, and contact with the eyes should be avoided. Neither is contraindicated in pregnancy or breastfeeding, although the manufacturers of selenium sulphide shampoo advise against its use during the first trimester of pregnancy. Selenium sulphide preparations are not recommended for children under 5 years of age.

Products

- Pyrithione zinc
  - Polytar AF shampoo (contains 1% pyrithione zinc with coal tar extracts and cade oil; it is the only licensed medicine to contain pyrithione zinc)
    Stiefel
  - Pyrithione zinc is included in several 'medicated' shampoos which are not licensed as medicines, including Head and Shoulders
    Procter & Gamble (HB&C)

- Selenium sulphide
  - Selsun shampoo (2.5%)
    Chattem

Ketoconazole

Mode of action

Ketoconazole is available as a 2% shampoo. It is an azole antifungal, which inhibits replication of yeast cells by interfering with the synthesis of ergosterol – a vital component of the cell membrane. Studies have shown ketoconazole to be effective in clearing dandruff and scalp seborrhoea; it is more effective than pyrithione zinc and about as effective as selenium sulphide, although ketoconazole appears to be better tolerated.[2-4] Ketoconazole shampoo is more expensive than selenium sulphide and 'medicated' pyrithione zinc preparations.

Administration

To clear dandruff and seborrhoeic dermatitis, the shampoo is used twice weekly for 2–4 weeks; it should be left on the hair for 3–5 minutes on each application. The condition can then be controlled with weekly or fortnightly use.

Contraindications, cautions and side-effects

Ketoconazole shampoo appears to be extremely safe to use. The compound has not been detected in plasma following topical use, and the shampoo does not cause the adverse effects and interactions associated with systemic use. Skin irritation has been reported only very rarely. It is not contraindicated in pregnancy.

Products

- Dandrazol antidandruff shampoo
  Transdermal

- Nizoral dandruff shampoo
  McNeil

Coal tar and other tar products

A wide range of products is licensed for dandruff, seborrhoeic dermatitis and psoriasis of the scalp, and available without prescription. Most of these products contain combinations of ingredients, of which coal tar is the most popular.

Mode of action

The mode of action of coal tar is unclear; it does not appear to reduce cell proliferation but appears to prevent the formation of squames or flakes of dandruff by interfering with the formation of intracellular cement. It also appears to impede the formation of sebum, and to have antipruritic properties.

Products

At least a dozen formulations are available for use on the hair, containing different coal tar solutions and extracts in varying concentrations, often in association with other tar derivatives and other constituents. The rationale for these combinations is unclear, as there is little evidence for synergistic or additive effects of constituents in the treatment of dandruff. Concerns have recently arisen over possible carcinogenicity and mutagenicity of coal tar, and special precautions for handling the raw material are now required; so far, however, no restrictions have been placed on the use of manufactured products.

Some examples of preparations that contain coal tar are:

- Alphosyl 2 in 1 shampoo
  GSK Consumer Healthcare

- Clinitar shampoo
  Cambridge Healthcare Supplies

- Pentrax shampoo
  Alliance

- Polytar liquid
  Stiefel

Keratolytic agents

The keratolytic properties and possible adverse effects of salicylic acid are described in the chapters on Athlete's foot and Acne.

Mode of action

In the treatment of dandruff, salicylic acid, at adequate concentration, would be expected to help break up dandruff squames and loosen them from the scalp.

Administration

Three proprietary shampoos containing salicylic acid (in combination with other constituents), at concentrations varying from 0.5 to 3%, are licensed for the treatment of dandruff, seborrhoeic dermatitis and other scaly conditions of the scalp. A minimum concentration of 1% is reported to be necessary to show a keratolytic effect on the scalp, but a prolonged contact time is needed and the effect takes up to 10 days to develop. Shampoos containing salicylic acid are greatly diluted on application, contact time is minimal and there is unlikely to be sufficient left on the scalp after rinsing to exert a residual effect, casting doubt on their effectiveness. Nevertheless, a trial found that a shampoo containing 3% salicylic acid was as effective in controlling dandruff as Nizoral (2% ketoconazole).[5] Some shampoos contain other keratolytic agents, including sulphur, which is believed to increase sloughing of cells via an inflammatory process, and allantoin, which is claimed to have chemical debriding properties.

One ointment containing salicylic acid and coal tar is available; it is likely to be more effective than shampoos but is messy to use and the risk of adverse effects is greater.

Products

- Capasal therapeutic shampoo
  Dermal

- Meted shampoo
  Alliance

- Cocois coconut oil compound
  Celltech

Antimicrobial detergents

Ceanel Concentrate (Ferndale) contains cetrimide, a quaternary ammonium antiseptic and cationic surfactant, together with an anti-fungal agent, undecenoic acid, at very low concentration. It may be no more effective against dandruff than regular use of an ordinary shampoo.

- Pyrithione zinc, selenium sulphide and ketoconazole shampoos are all effective in controlling dandruff. Ketoconazole appears to be more effective than pyrithione zinc but not selenium sulphide, although the latter is less pleasant to use. Ketoconazole shampoo is more expensive than shampoos containing either of the other two compounds.
- Only one product containing pyrithione zinc is licensed as a medicine, but several brands and own-label versions are available as 'medicated' shampoos.
- A wide range of shampoos containing coal tar, keratolytic agents and microbial detergents is available. They have been traditionally used for dandruff and there appears to be general satisfaction with their performance; however, there is little clinical evidence of their effectiveness.

PRODUCT RECOMMENDATIONS

Regular (twice weekly) use of an ordinary shampoo should be tried initially. If this is not effective, the treatments of choice appear to be:

- ketoconazole (on grounds of efficacy but not cost)
- selenium sulphide (on grounds of efficacy and cost but not cosmetic acceptability)
- a 'medicated' pyrithione zinc shampoo (on grounds of cost and cosmetic acceptability).

However, clinicians and patients also seem satisfied with coal-tar-based preparations.

REFERENCES

1. Orentreich N, Taylor EH, Berger RA, Auerbach R. Comparative study of two antidandruff preparations. *J Pharm Sci* 1969; 58: 1279–1280.

2. Pierard-Franchimont C, Goffin V, Decroix J, Pierard GE. A multicenter randomized trial of ketoconazole 2% and zinc pyrithione 1% shampoos in severe dandruff and seborrheic dermatitis. *Skin Pharmacol Appl Skin Physiol* 2002; 15: 434–441.

3. Peter RU, Richarz-Barthauer U. Successful treatment and prophylaxis of scalp seborrhoeic dermatitis and dandruff with 2% ketoconazole shampoo: results of a multicentre, double-blind, placebo-controlled trial. *Br J Dermatol* 1995; 132: 441–445.

4. Danby FW, Maddin WS, Margesson LJ, Rosenthal D. A randomized, double-blind, placebo-controlled trial of ketoconazole 2% shampoo versus selenium sulfide 2.5% shampoo in the treatment of moderate to severe dandruff. *J Am Acad Dermatol* 1993; 29: 1008–1012.

5. Squire RA, Goode K. A randomised, single-blind, single-centre clinical trial to evaluate comparative clinical efficacy of shampoos containing ciclopirox olamine (1.5%) and salicylic acid (3%), or ketoconazole (2%, Nizoral) for the treatment of dandruff/seborrhoeic dermatitis. *J Dermatolog Treat* 2002; 13: 51–60.

Diarrhoea

Diarrhoea of an acute self-limiting nature can be treated with non-prescription medicines.

CAUSES

Diarrhoea of the acute self-limiting type is generally caused by either bacterial or viral infection through ingestion of contaminated food or drink. Some bacteria (e.g. toxigenic *Escherichia coli* and *Staphylococcus aureus*) produce toxins that bind to the mucosal cells of the small intestine, causing hypersecretion of fluid. This overwhelms the reabsorbing capacity of the colon and results in watery diarrhoea, often with little or no fever or other symptoms. Other bacteria (e.g. invasive *E. coli*, *Salmonella* and *Shigella*) directly invade mucosal epithelial cells and cause an inflammatory reaction, producing diarrhoea that is less fluid but accompanied by nausea, vomiting, cramps and sometimes low-grade fever. Viral infections, which often affect babies and young children, also produce watery diarrhoea. Acute diarrhoea can also have non-infective causes, such as stress, alcohol and hot, spicy food.

Normal faeces contain 60–85% water, and 70–200 mL water per day is lost from the body through defecation. In diarrhoea, water loss of up to four times this volume per loose stool occurs, and sodium and potassium alkaline salts are excreted along with it, leading to a fall in plasma pH (acidosis), which can have serious metabolic consequences. Fluid and electrolyte losses are increased further if vomiting also occurs.

The situation is especially hazardous in babies and young children, as a relatively high proportion of total body weight is lost, and dehydration can occur very rapidly. The elderly are also particularly sensitive to the effects of fluid and electrolyte loss, especially if they are taking diuretics. Reduction in blood volume resulting from excessive loss of fluid through diarrhoea may stimulate the secretion of aldosterone from the adrenal cortex, causing excretion of potassium and leading to hypokalaemia. Excessive fluid loss may also lead to renal failure through reduction of renal artery blood flow.

TREATMENT

Guidelines for treatment of diarrhoea are inconsistent and sometimes contradictory. One point of view is to regard diarrhoea as the natural way to 'flush out' the causative organisms and toxins from the bowel, and the use of antidiarrhoeals, which are either intestinal antimotility agents or adsorbents, is considered unnecessary and sometimes undesirable. On the other hand, it is recognised that sufferers often wish to curtail diarrhoea for reasons of comfort or convenience, and there is no evidence that this is neither safe nor prolongs the illness.[1] However, treatment with antimotility agents or adsorbents should be as adjunctive therapy to appropriate rehydration. Before recommending any treatment, serious underlying causes of diarrhoea must be considered and excluded. In addition, referral should be made for any episode lasting more than 72 hours in adults and older children, 48 hours in children under 3 years of age and the elderly, and 24 hours in children under 1 year of age. Infants under 3 months of age should be referred immediately.

Oral rehydration therapy

Fluid and electrolyte replacement by oral rehydration therapy (ORT) is generally regarded as the first line of treatment for acute diarrhoea, despite a lack of directly relevant evidence. There appear to be no systematic reviews or randomised controlled trials evaluating the effects of oral rehydration solutions for acute diarrhoea relevant to people living in developed countries such as the UK, although ORT has been shown to be beneficial for treating diarrhoea in people living in developing countries.[2] ORT is particularly important for the very young and the elderly.

Mode of action

Oral rehydration salts (ORS) are designed to replace water and electrolytes lost through diarrhoea and vomiting, but they are not intended to relieve symptoms. They contain sodium and potassium salts to replace these essential ions, and citrate and/or bicarbonate to correct acidosis. Glucose is also an important ingredient, as it acts as a carrier for the transport of sodium ions, and hence water, across the mucosa of the small intestine.

The composition of the ORS preparations available in the UK varies between products, but all are designed to correct fluid loss and electrolyte imbalance associated with mild-to-moderate diarrhoea. The sodium content is in the range 50–60 mmol/L and the glucose content up to 200 mmol/L. World Health Organization ORS contain a higher concentration of sodium (75 mmol/L), and are intended for use mainly in developing countries where conditions causing severe diarrhoea and fluid loss are relatively common.

ORT is not intended to stop diarrhoea, but acute diarrhoea is self-limiting and normally ceases within 24–48 hours. ORT can be recommended for patients of any age, even when referral to a doctor is considered necessary.

An oral rehydration product (Dioralyte Relief, Sanofi-Aventis) containing powdered rice starch in place of glucose is claimed to achieve even greater rehydration than glucose over time, and the rice starch is claimed to help produce firmer stools, leading to faster recovery compared with glucose. A Cochrane Review[3] found that the product was effective in reducing stool output and consequent fluid loss in people suffering from cholera, but that it had little effect in infants and children with non-cholera diarrhoea.

Dosage and administration

The contents of one sachet of ORS should be dissolved in 200 mL water; for infants the water should be freshly boiled and cooled. It is important to make up the solution exactly to the recommended volume, as too concentrated a solution will be hyperosmolar, drawing more water into the intestine and exacerbating the diarrhoea and dehydration. To avoid risk of possible exposure to further infection, the solution should be discarded not later than 1 hour after reconstitution, or it may be kept for up to 24 hours if stored in a refrigerator.

The recommended dose of ORS for an adult is 200–400 mL after every loose motion, or 2–4 L over 4–6 hours. (Diabetic patients can use ORS, but they should be reminded to monitor blood glucose levels carefully.) Patients may prefer to sip one or two teaspoonfuls every few minutes rather than drink large quantities less frequently. Children over 2 years of age should be offered a cupful (200 mL) of solution after each loose stool; children under 2 years of age should be offered quarter–half a cupful. Infants should be given one to one-and-a-half times the normal feed volume. Both breastfed and formula-fed babies should be fed normally during diarrhoea; formula feed should not be diluted.

Contraindications and cautions

There are no contraindications to ORT unless the patient is vomiting frequently and unable to keep the solution down, in which case intravenous fluid and electrolyte replacement may be necessary. Fluid overload from excessive administration of ORS is highly unlikely, but is possible if it is continued in babies and young children for more than 48 hours. Fluid overload is recognised by the eyelids becoming puffy, and is rapidly corrected by withholding ORS and other liquids.

Products

- Dioralyte sachets and tablets
  Sanofi-Aventis

- Dioralyte Relief sachets
  Sanofi-Aventis

- Electrolade sachets
  Thornton & Ross

Opioids

Compounds available

The following compounds are available:

- loperamide
- morphine
- codeine
- diphenoxylate (in co-phenotrope).

Mode of action

One of the effects of morphine and the opioid drugs is to cause constipation by increasing the tone of both the small and large bowel and reducing intestinal motility. These drugs also increase sphincter tone and decrease secretory activity along the gastrointestinal tract. Decreased motility enhances fluid and electrolyte reabsorption and decreases the volume of intestinal contents.

Loperamide has a high affinity for, and exerts a direct action on, opiate receptors in the gut wall. It also undergoes extensive first-pass metabolism so very little reaches the systemic circulation; it is unlikely to cause any of the side-effects associated with opiates at the restricted dosage permitted for non-prescription use. Several controlled trials[2] have shown it to be effective in reducing the duration of diarrhoea, although it should be remembered that acute diarrhoea is in any case self-limiting and relatively short-lived.

Morphine acts promptly on the intestine (within 1 hour of administration) because of its direct action on intestinal smooth muscle and quick absorption from the gastrointestinal tract. Its action peaks within 2–3 hours and lasts about 4 hours. Morphine is not well absorbed orally and in combination products its availability may be reduced because of adsorption onto other constituents.

Codeine is a weaker opioid than morphine. It is a constituent of Kaodene (Sovereign), the recommended dose of which contains 20 mg codeine. (The *British National Formulary* recommends a dose of 30 mg for the treatment of acute diarrhoea and a range of 15–60 mg.)

Diphenoxylate is a synthetic derivative of pethidine. It has little or no central action but acts selectively on gastrointestinal smooth muscle. Diphenoxylate is available in combination with atropine as co-phenotrope (diphenoxylate hydrochloride 2.5 mg/atropine 25 micrograms). Atropine is included at a subtherapeutic dose to discourage abuse of the opioid, on the premise that unpleasant antimuscarinic effects will be experienced if higher-than-recommended doses are taken. There appears to be little evidence of the effectiveness of co-phenotrope, but one randomised controlled trial found that it significantly reduced the rate of bowel actions compared with placebo, although it did not actually reduce the duration of diarrhoea.[4]

Dosage

The dose of loperamide capsules for adults and children over 12 years is 4 mg initially, followed by 2 mg after each loose bowel movement, up to a maximum of eight capsules (16 mg) in 24 hours. If symptoms have not subsided within 24 hours, the patient should be referred. Loperamide is not licensed for non-prescription use in children under 12 years of age, and should not be recommended to pregnant or breastfeeding women.

The morphine content per recommended dose of the products listed below ranges between 0.5 and 1 mg. The effectiveness of these small amounts in controlling diarrhoea is debatable; no specific effective dose has been stated by the UK authorities, but the US Food and Drug Administration considers morphine doses in the range 1.5–2 mg to be effective.

The dosage of co-phenotrope is, for adults and adolescents over 16 years of age, four tablets initially, followed by two tablets every 6 hours, to a maximum of 10 tablets in 24 hours. Patients should be referred if symptoms persist after treatment for 24 hours.

Side-effects and cautions

The use of opioids as antidiarrhoeals is limited by their actions on the central nervous system (CNS), which include CNS depression and the risk of dependence. However, the risk of dependence at usual dosages for acute diarrhoeal episodes is low. Community pharmacists will, none-the-less, be well aware of the abuse potential of over-the-counter products containing morphine and codeine.

Products

- Loperamide (several brands are available)
- Loperamide with simeticone (Imodium Plus, McNeil)

Loperamide (2 mg) is formulated with the surfactant compound simeticone (125 mg) in a chewable tablet. The manufacturers claim that the combined formulation relieves the cramping and bloating that can accompany diarrhoea, and that it improves the effectiveness of loperamide. A study carried out by the manufacturers[5] involving nearly 500 patients has shown that the combination product considerably reduced the duration of diarrhoea and relieved gas-related discomfort in comparison with loperamide alone. The dosage of this product is two tablets initially for adults over 18 years of age (one tablet for young adults aged 12–18 years) followed by one tablet after each loose stool (for all ages from 12 years). The maximum dosage is four tablets daily for 2 days.

- Loperamide with rehydration salts
  - Diocalm Complete (loperamide capsules packaged together with oral rehydration salts sachets)
    SSL International

- Morphine (licensed for use in adults and children from the age of 6 years)
  - Kaolin and Morphine Mixture BP
  - J. Collis Browne's mixture and tablets
    Thornton & Ross
  - Diocalm Dual Action tablets (also contains attapulgite)
    SSL International

— Opazimes tablets (also contains aluminium hydroxide, kaolin and belladonna dry extract)
  Co-Pharma

- Codeine
  — Kaodene (contains 10 mg codeine phosphate and 3 g kaolin in 10 mL – licensed for use in adults and children from the age of 5 years)
  Sovereign

- Diphenoxylate (in co-phenotrope)
  — Dymotil
  Goldshield

Adsorbents

The following compounds are available:

- kaolin
- pectin
- attapulgite
- bismuth subsalicylate.

Kaolin is a natural hydrated aluminium silicate that has been used in the treatment of diarrhoea since ancient Greek times. It is not absorbed from the gastrointestinal tract, and about 90% of the drug is metabolised in the gut and excreted in the faeces.

Pectin is a purified carbohydrate obtained from the rind of citrus fruit or pomace (crushed apple); its mode of action is uncertain.

Attapulgite is a naturally occurring clay mineral, consisting of hydrous magnesium aluminium silicate. Its adsorptive capacity can be increased by thermal treatment; the heat-treated form is known as activated attapulgite. *In vitro* alkaloidal adsorptive studies have shown activated attapulgite to have an adsorptive capacity for certain toxic compounds that is five times greater than that of kaolin. Both kaolin and attapulgite have varying and relatively weak adsorptive properties in respect of diarrhoea-producing bacteria. In a small, double-blind, placebo-controlled study,[6] attapulgite was significantly better than placebo in reducing the severity and duration of diarrhoea in terms of frequency of motion, consistency of stools and severity of dehydration and in reducing the amount of ORS consumed. However, in a parallel open-label study,[7] attapulgite was significantly less effective at controlling diarrhoea symptoms than loperamide.

Attapulgite and activated attapulgite are contained in one product: Diocalm Dual Action.

Bismuth subsalicylate is claimed to possess adsorbent properties, and some studies have shown it to be effective in treating diarrhoea.[8–10] Large doses are required, however, and salicylate absorption may occur. It should therefore be avoided by individuals sensitive to aspirin.

Mode of action

The rationale behind the use of adsorbents is that they are capable of adsorbing microbial toxins and microorganisms onto their surfaces. Because the drugs are not absorbed from the gastrointestinal tract, adsorbed toxins and microorganisms are ultimately excreted in the stool. In addition, adsorbents, particularly hydrophilic organic polymers (e.g. pectin and bulk-forming agents), bind water within the intestine, causing watery stools to become more formed. Bulk-forming agents (e.g. ispaghula, methylcellulose and sterculia), which are plant-derived polysaccharide products that absorb water and add bulk to stools, are used to treat some forms of chronic diarrhoea. They are more usually used as laxatives (see chapter on Constipation).

Adsorbents are used as the main constituents in antidiarrhoeal preparations for young children, in whom opioids are contraindicated. As they are largely unabsorbed from the intestine, adsorbents are relatively harmless and safe to use, but there is little evidence that they are effective. It has also been argued that if they do reduce evacuation of faeces, they may prolong the presence of offending pathogens and toxins in the bowel. Adsorption is a non-specific process and as well as adsorbing toxins, bacteria and water, the drugs may interfere with the absorption of other drugs from the intestine.

This should be borne in mind if recommending adsorbent antidiarrhoeals to patients taking other medicines.

Products

(See also products listed above under morphine and codeine.)

- Kaolin
  - Kaolin Mixture BP
  - Entrocalm tablets (also contains calcium carbonate)
    Galpharm International
  - Junior KaoC suspension (also contains calcium carbonate)
    Torbet

- Attapulgite (and activated attapulgite) (constituents of Diocalm Dual Action)
  SSL International

- Bismuth subsalicylate
  - Pepto-Bismol
    Procter & Gamble

Belladonna

Belladonna dry extract is a constituent of Opazimes (Co-Pharma) tablets, together with morphine, aluminium hydroxide and kaolin. The mode of action of belladonna extract, its contraindications and interactions are described under Antispasmodics in the chapter on Indigestion.

Mode of action

The function of belladonna in this product is presumably to reduce the frequency and force of movement of the smooth muscle of the intestine, in order to relieve pain and reduce the intensity of diarrhoea.

Dosage

Belladonna Dry Extract BP 1988 contains 1% alkaloids calculated as hyoscyamine, and the hyoscyamine content of the recommended dosage of Opazimes tablets is 60 micrograms. The recommended dose of hyoscyamine as an antispasmodic is 150–300 micrograms, and it would therefore appear that the content of belladonna dry extract in these products is subtherapeutic. In addition, belladonna dry extract is formulated together with morphine (0.5 mg per recommended dose), which directly opposes the effect of belladonna on intestinal tone, so the inclusion of both seems irrational from a pharmacological viewpoint.

PRODUCT SELECTION POINTS

- Acute infective diarrhoea is a self-limiting condition that normally resolves without treatment within a couple of days. It is debatable whether any attempt should be made to stop acute diarrhoea, although patients' desire not to suffer the discomfort and inconvenience it causes is understandable. If patients will accept the advice, the best course of action is to recommend ORT and provide reassurance.
- Patients should be referred to a doctor if diarrhoea persists for more than 24 hours in babies between 3 months and 1 year of age, for 2 days in children under 3 years and elderly patients, and 3 days in older children and adults. Babies under 3 months with diarrhoea should be referred immediately.
- The most important measure in managing acute diarrhoea is ensuring that the fluid and electrolytes lost are replaced and that dehydration is avoided. This is particularly important for elderly and very young patients.
- ORT can be safely recommended to any patient with diarrhoea, even if an antidiarrhoeal is also supplied or the patient has to be referred to a doctor.
- Loperamide or co-phenotrope are probably the most effective

non-prescription antidiarrhoeals, and are unlikely to cause any adverse effects at the recommended licensed dosages.

- Antidiarrhoeals containing morphine may not be very effective, given the low concentration of the drug in OTC products. Co-formulation with adsorbents may also reduce its availability. Morphine-containing products are liable to abuse.
- There is little evidence that adsorbents are effective as antidiarrhoeals, but they should do no harm. They can be given safely to younger children if a parent insists on wanting to stop the diarrhoea, although ORT should always be strongly recommended as well.
- The single product available that contains belladonna extract appears to have little value, given the low concentration of the drug. In addition, the combination of belladonna with morphine seems pharmacologically irrational.

PRODUCT RECOMMENDATIONS

Based on rational criteria, the choice of products available for diarrhoea is limited.

- ORT is the first-line treatment for all patients and in all circumstances, and particularly for babies, young children and the elderly.
- For adults who want to curtail diarrhoea – a loperamide preparation or co-phenotrope.

REFERENCES

1. Wingate D, Phillips SF, Lewis SJ, *et al.* Guidelines for adults on self-medication for the treatment of acute diarrhoea. *Aliment Pharmacol Ther* 2001; 15: 773–782.
2. *Clinical Evidence*. London: BMJ Publishing. (http://www.clinicalevidence.com/) (Accessed 14 July 2005).

3.   Fontaine O, Gore SM, Pierce NF. Rice-based oral rehydration solution for treating diarrhoea. *The Cochrane Library,* issue 2. Chichester, UK: John Wiley & Sons, 2000 (www.thecochranelibrary.com).

4.   Lustman F, Walters EG, Shroff NE, *et al.* Diphenoxylate hydrochloride (Lomotil) in the treatment of acute diarrhoea. *Br J Clin Pract* 1987; 41: 648–651.

5.   Kaplan MA, Prior MJ, Ash RR, *et al.* Loperamide-simethicone vs loperamide alone, simethicone alone, and placebo in the treatment of acute diarrhoea with gas-related abdominal discomfort. A randomized controlled trial. *Arch Fam Med* 1999; 8: 243–248.

6.   Zaid MR, Hasan M, Khan AA. Attapulgite in the treatment of acute diarrhoea: a double-blind placebo-controlled study. *J Diarrhoeal Dis Res* 1995; 13: 44–46.

7.   DuPont HL, Ericsson CD, DuPont MW, *et al.* A randomized, open-label comparison of nonprescription loperamide and attapulgite in the symptomatic treatment of acute diarrhea. *Am J Med* 1990; 88: 20S–23S.

8.   Du Pont HL. Bismuth subsalicylate in the treatment and prevention of diarrheal disease. *Drug Intell Clin Pharm* 1987; 21: 687–693.

9.   Du Pont HL, Sullivan P, Pickering LK. Symptomatic treatment of diarrhoea with bismuth subsalicylate. *Gastroenterology* 1977; 73: 715–718.

10. Ericsson CD, Du Pont HL, Johnson PC. Non-antibiotic therapy for travellers' diarrhoea. *Rev Infect Dis* 1986; 8 (Suppl. 2): S202–S206.

Dry skin

Dry skin is a common condition that nearly everybody experiences at some time.

CAUSES

Dry skin results from inadequate moisture content in the stratum corneum. It is associated with a range of skin conditions, including contact dermatitis, atopic eczema and psoriasis, and with various systemic disorders such as hypothyroidism, arthritis and autoimmune conditions.

Dry skin becomes more common with increasing age because of thinning of the epidermis and its reduced ability to retain moisture. In healthy people, dehydration of the skin may be caused by cold weather, over-exposure to the sun or by occupational exposure to dehydrating agents.

The symptoms of dry skin include roughness and flaking, loss of flexibility, fissures, hyperkeratosis, inflammation and pruritus, in varying degrees of severity depending on the cause and individual response; they appear when the water content of the stratum corneum falls below 10%.

TREATMENT

The principle of treatment for dry skin is rehydration of the stratum corneum to its normal level of 10–20%. Moisturising and emollient preparations are formulated to achieve this by replacing water lost from the epidermis (although this is only possible to a limited extent) and by preventing further evaporation. The latter may be achieved simply by applying a film of oil to the skin while it is wet or directly after it has been wetted and dried, for example by adding oil to a bath or applying it directly afterwards. However, for minor dry-skin conditions, oil-in-water emulsions provide a more aesthetically acceptable method.

Emulsions first hydrate the skin, various constituents being used to enhance water penetration or uptake by the epidermis (see below).

Loss of water from the emulsion, mainly by evaporation and to a lesser extent by absorption into the skin, in addition to the mechanical stress caused by its application, then causes the emulsion to crack, releasing the oil phase. The layer of oil forms a hydrophobic seal over the skin, which retards further water evaporation.

Oil-in-water creams and lotions also have a cosmetic effect through smoothing down the rough, scaly surface of dry skin and reducing mechanical drag, making it feel smooth to the touch. Water evaporation, especially from emollients with a higher water content, produces a cooling effect on the skin, which alleviates the pruritus that accompanies dry-skin conditions such as eczema.

The degree of occlusiveness and prevention of water evaporation depends on the oil content of an emulsion. Water-in-oil preparations with a very greasy texture are also available; these may be suitable for more severe dry-skin and eczematous conditions but are generally less aesthetically acceptable for use in mild dry-skin conditions.

A wide range of proprietary emollient products is available in a variety of presentations, including creams, ointments, lotions, bath oils, water-dispersible bath additives, an aerosol spray and a shower gel. Although some are expensive and usually supplied on prescription, all can be bought over the counter. There are also some inexpensive formulary emollient preparations, including Emulsifying Ointment BP and Aqueous Cream BP, which consists of 30% emulsifying ointment with water. These may be as effective as more expensive products, although less cosmetically elegant than some. There has been some controversy over the appropriateness of using Aqueous Cream BP purely on the grounds of cheapness: the Skin Care Campaign, an alliance of groups including UK national dermatology patient organisations and health professionals, has expressed concern that it causes sensitisation in substantial numbers of people, particularly children.[1] Sensitisation has been ascribed to the partitioning of the emulsifying agent, sodium lauryl sulphate, in the formulation.

With such a wide choice of products and little objective evidence of relative effectiveness, choice is often a matter of personal preference.[2,3]

Emollient preparations are generally very safe to use, the only contraindication being sensitivity to constituents. The principal constituents of emollient products are reviewed below.

Paraffins

Hard, soft and liquid paraffins are mixtures of hydrocarbons obtained from petroleum; liquid paraffin is also known as mineral oil. Soft and liquid paraffins can be used on their own as emollients and are effective occlusive agents. However, they are usually not cosmetically acceptable as they are greasy and difficult to wash off the skin, and their occlusive effects can sometimes lead to maceration of the skin, which may aggravate existing dermatitis. Mixtures of hard, soft and liquid paraffins are used as bases in many emollient and other dermatological creams.

Product examples

- Aqueous Cream BP
- Emulsifying Ointment BP
- Alpha Keri bath oil
  Bristol-Myers Squibb

- Cetraben Emollient bath additive
  Sankyo

- Diprobase cream
  Schering-Plough

- Diprobath bath additive
  Schering-Plough

- E45 cream
  Crookes

- Oilatum cream and bath formula
  Stiefel

- Ultrabase cream
  Schering Health

- Unguentum M cream
  Crookes

Glycerol, propylene glycol and sodium pidolate

Glycerol is a trihydric alcohol; it is hygroscopic and is included in emollient and hydrating products to promote the retention of water in the skin. It also improves the feel and consistency of formulations, making them more pleasant to use. Propylene glycol and sodium pidolate have hygroscopic properties similar to glycerol; they are used in emollients to increase hydration of the skin.

Product examples

- Hydromol cream
  Ferndale

- LactiCare lotion
  Stiefel

- Neutrogena Norwegian Formula dermatological cream
  Neutrogena

- Probase 3 cream
  Schering-Plough

Urea

At a concentration of 10%, urea increases hydration of the skin. (At higher concentrations, it is claimed to have keratolytic and antipruritic properties.) Urea can cause burning or stinging, and may irritate inflamed skin, but this is usually minimised by formulating products to a pH of 6.

Product examples

- Aquadrate cream
  Alliance

- Calmurid cream
  Galderma

Both of the above contain 10% urea.

Lactic acid

Lactic acid and other alpha-hydroxy acids increase hydration of the skin and control keratinisation.

Product examples

- Calmurid
  Galderma

- LactiCare lotion
  Stiefel

Natural products

Lanolin (anhydrous wool fat) is derived from the sebum of sheep and is thought to be similar to human sebum. It is an excellent emollient, being highly water absorbent (up to about 30%) and therefore a useful water-in-oil emulsifier. It is also occlusive. Lanolin has become less popular as an emollient in recent years because of reports of sensitisation, but purified and hypoallergenic derivatives have been developed and it is still included in several products.

Isopropyl myristate is a fatty acid ester derived from coconut oil. It is included as an ingredient in several emollients, being stable in formulations, fairly readily absorbed into the skin and having a good 'skin feel'. Soya and almond oils are also used in emollient products.

Product examples

- Balneum bath treatment
  Crookes

- Dermol 500 lotion
  Dermal

- Diprobath bath additive
  Schering-Plough

- Emulsiderm emollient emulsion
  Dermal

- Hydromol cream
  Ferndale

- Imuderm therapeutic oil
  Goldshield Healthcare

Administration

Treatment regimens depend on the condition, and can range from daily baths containing oils or emollient additives followed by liberal application of further emollients, to the occasional application of a cream to a patch of dry skin. Patients needing the former are likely to be under medical supervision, but pharmacists should be able to advise them on how to use products to best effect.

A bath is good therapy for atopic eczema or severe dry skin as it hydrates the skin and provides a good base for the application of emollients. Between 10 and 30 mL bath additive (the exact amount depends on the product) should be added to a lukewarm bath (at about 37°C). (Water that is too hot will cause dilation of the blood vessels and can make the itching of eczema worse.) Emulsifying Ointment BP can be used as a bath additive: about 30 g should be whisked up with hot water in a jug and then poured under the running water. After bathing, the skin should be patted, not rubbed, dry.

Hydration is claimed to increase the efficacy of topical medication tenfold, so an emollient should be applied immediately, before the skin dries out.

Emollients are safe to use and can be applied as frequently as needed during the day. For patients with atopic eczema, the emollient can be applied liberally over the entire body, including the face and scalp if needed.

PRODUCT SELECTION POINTS

- A wide range of emollient products is available in a variety of presentations, although some are intended primarily for use in atopic eczema and chronic dry-skin conditions. Oil-in-water creams or lotions are generally the most suitable and cosmetically acceptable preparations for mild dry-skin conditions.
- With little evidence of comparative effectiveness, choice is generally based on personal preference and cost.

PRODUCT RECOMMENDATIONS

- For mild dry-skin conditions – an oil-in-water emollient cream or lotion.
- For atopic eczema and chronic dry-skin conditions – emollients, the choice of product and presentation depending on the situation and individual preference.

REFERENCES

1. Aqueous cream may be "cheap" but is it always appropriate? *Pharm J* 2000; 265: 325.
2. Clarke C, Hoare C. Making the most of emollients. *Pharm J* 2001; 266: 227–229.
3. Hoare C, Li Wan Po A, Williams H. Systematic review of treatments for atopic eczema. *Health Technol Assess* 2000; 4(37).

Ear problems

Ear problems offer little scope for pharmacists to advise on treatment, as patients' descriptions of their symptoms and their own self-diagnoses may be misleading; medical examination is usually necessary for accurate diagnosis.

Earache

In adults, earache may sometimes be associated with an upper respiratory tract infection, and, as long as the pain is not severe, can be treated with oral analgesics for up to 48 hours, before referral if the condition does not improve. Earache in children should always be referred, as otitis media is fairly common and repeated attacks can lead to permanent damage if not managed properly; use of an oral analgesic can be advised until a doctor can be seen. Analgesic ear drops are available without prescription but are not generally recommended.

Ear wax

Cerumen (ear wax) is a complex oily fluid secreted by sebaceous and apocrine glands in the external auditory canal, which combines with exfoliated skin cells to form a protective waxy layer. This is normally moved outwards by movement of the jaw in speaking and chewing, and removed by washing. In some individuals, however, excessive cohesive cerumen is produced. This forms a waxy plug that affects hearing and causes discomfort. The prophylactic use of a cerumenolytic preparation is sometimes recommended. Generally, however, syringing is necessary to remove ear wax, although cerumenolytics can be used in advance to soften, loosen and partially dissolve the wax.

Otitis externa

Otitis externa is inflammation of the external auditory canal. The acute form is usually caused by bacterial infection, but may also be fungal or viral. The chronic form is eczematous and may be atopic or a contact dermatitis. Dermatitis may become infected and the two types of otitis externa can exist together.

TREATMENT

Earache

Compound/product available

Only one formulation that contains an analgesic constituent – choline salicylate – is available without prescription; the product also contains glycerol. It is available as two brands – Audax and Earex Plus (both SSL International) and is licensed for the relief of earache and softening of ear wax.

Mode of action

Choline salicylate is used as a local analgesic (it is also included in gels for the treatment of sore mouths and mouth ulcers). It has a counterirritant effect, and is also hydrolysed by cutaneous esterases to produce salicylic acid, which probably exerts some anti-inflammatory effect by blocking prostaglandin formation. One small double-blind trial found Audax ear drops to be more effective than placebo as an analgesic.[1] However, the *British National Formulary* states that choline salicylate is of doubtful value when applied topically.

Audax and Earex Plus also contain glycerol, and in a comparative trial[2] Audax was found to be a more efficient cerumenolytic than Earex drops (although not significantly), another brand marketed by the same company that contains fixed and volatile oils. Glycerol has been claimed to be as effective as anything else for softening ear wax.

Although marketed as cerumenolytics and not for the relief of
ear pain, some other brands of ear drops contain constituents with
counterirritant or local analgesic properties, such as camphor oil,
chlorbutol, turpentine oil and terpineol, which may have some analgesic effects.

Ear wax

Although cerumenolytic ear drops for the softening of ear wax are
available, they should generally only be supplied if a doctor or a nurse
trained to diagnose ear conditions has advised their use, as patients
often mistakenly ascribe any ear problem, including loss of hearing,
discomfort and pain, to ear wax.

Cerumenolytics may soften ear wax and make it easier to
remove by syringing, but are unlikely to dissolve and remove com-
pacted plugs on their own.

Several approaches are taken to loosening and dissolving wax in
the ear, including the use of aqueous and oily solvents and surfactants,
and oxygen generation to facilitate penetration of water into the plug.
Constituents of cerumenolytic products include fixed and volatile oils,
glycerol, docusate, urea hydrogen peroxide and paradichlorobenzene.
However, ear-wax-softening agents have been found to be no more
effective than using warm water or saline shortly before syringing.[3,4]
In general, little difference in efficacy between cerumenolytics has
been found, although trials to date have been of poor quality.[5,6]

Constituents of cerumenolytic ear drops

- **Fixed and volatile oils:** As wax contains a high proportion of
  oily components, it is logical to assume that it can be dissolved,
  at least partially, by oils. The *British National Formulary* recommends the use of olive oil or almond oil to soften wax before
  removal. Earex ear drops (SSL International) contain arachis,
  almond and camphor oils in equal proportions.
- **Docusate sodium** is a surface active agent that increases water

penetration into the wax plug. Molcer ear drops (Wallace) contain 5% docusate sodium; Waxsol ear drops (Norgine) originally contained this concentration but were reformulated in the mid-1980s to a content of 0.5% following reports of local irritation.

- **Urea hydrogen peroxide:** Exterol (Dermal) and Otex (Dendron) ear drops both contain 5% urea hydrogen peroxide in a glycerol base. In contact with tissues containing the enzyme catalase, hydrogen peroxide releases its oxygen to create effervescence, which helps to break up wax by a mechanical action. The glycerol assists in softening the wax; the urea increases penetration of the solution into the plug. Hydrogen Peroxide Solution BP 20 volume (6%), diluted one part with three parts water, can also be used but may not penetrate so effectively.
- **Sodium Bicarbonate Ear Drops BP** contains 5% sodium bicarbonate and 30% glycerol in water, and is recommended in the *British National Formulary*.
- **Paradichlorobenzene** is contained in Cerumol ear drops (LAB), in an oily base with chlorbutanol, which it is claimed assists the oil to penetrate ear-wax plugs.

Administration of cerumenolytic ear drops

The following technique is recommended for the most effective use of ear drops.

- It is best to have another person instil the ear drops.
- Before use, the drops should be slightly warmed by holding in the hands for a few minutes.
- The patient should lay their head on a flat surface such as a table, with the affected ear uppermost.
- The auricle (pinna) should be lifted upwards and backwards in adults, or downward and backwards in children, to straighten the ear canal.
- The requisite number of drops should be instilled.
- The tragus (the small projection in front of the external opening)

should be pressed gently once or twice, to assist the drops down the ear canal and to expel air bubbles.

- The patient should remain with their head down for at least 5 minutes. A cotton-wool plug moistened with the drops should be placed into the ear.
- Unless directed otherwise, the drops should be used night and morning for 3 or 4 days before syringing.

Otitis externa

Hydrocortisone cream

Mild eczematous otitis externa affecting the pinna can be treated with hydrocortisone cream. (For details, see chapter on Irritant and allergic dermatitis.)

Aluminium acetate

Aluminium acetate is astringent, hygroscopic and produces an acidic environment that is hostile to pathogenic bacteria. Aluminium Acetate (13%) Ear Drops BP can be used as an anti-inflammatory for eczematous otitis externa in the external ear canal. However, it is not readily available and may have to be obtained from a specials manufacturer, making it prohibitively expensive for over-the-counter sale.

Acetic acid

Acetic acid has antibacterial activity, and is reported to be active against *Haemophilus*, *Pseudomonas*, *Candida* and *Trichomonas* species. A 2% solution of acetic acid is available as a pump-action spray (EarCalm Spray [GSK Consumer Healthcare]), licensed for the treatment of superficial infections of the external auditory canal in adults and children over the age of 12 years. It is used 3–8 times daily until 2 days after symptoms have disappeared, for up to a maximum of 7 days. Use should be discontinued and medical advice sought if symptoms do not improve within 48 hours of starting treatment.

PRODUCT SELECTION POINTS

- Analgesic ear drops should not be recommended for earache unless the cause is known with certainty, and known not to be serious. Earache from an unknown cause should be treated with oral analgesics until a doctor can be seen.
- Cerumenolytic ear drops should not be recommended unless the presence of ear wax has been identified.
- There is no conclusive evidence that any cerumenolytic preparation is more effective than others. Instilling warm water or saline into the ear for a few minutes before syringing may be just as effective as wax-softening ear drops.

PRODUCT RECOMMENDATIONS

- For earache – oral analgesics only until a medical diagnosis is made.
- For ear wax (confirmed as such) – sodium bicarbonate ear drops are cheap and probably as effective as anything else. The *British National Formulary* considers that proprietary cerumenolytics should not be first choice.
- For mild eczematous otitis externa on the pinna – hydrocortisone cream.
- For mild infective otitis externa (confirmed as such) – acetic acid 2% solution.

REFERENCES

1. Hewitt HR. Clinical evaluation of choline salicylate ear drops. *Practitioner* 1970; 204: 438–441.
2. Lyndon S, Roy P, Grillage MG, Miller AJ. A comparison of the efficacy of two ear drop preparations ('Audax' and 'Earex') in the softening and removal of impacted ear wax. *Curr Med Res Opin* 1992; 13: 21–25.
3. Eekhof JA, de Bock GH, Le Cessie S, Springer MP. A quasi-randomised controlled trial of water as a quick softening agent of persistent earwax in general practice. *Br J Gen Pract* 2001; 51: 635–637.

4.   Whatley VN, Dodds CL, Paul RI. Randomized clinical trial of docusate, triethanolamine polypeptide, and irrigation in cerumen removal in children. *Arch Pediatr Adolesc Med* 2003; 157: 1177–1180.

5.   Burton MJ, Doree CJ. Ear drops for the removal of ear wax.*The Cochrane Library*, issue 3. Chichester, UK: John Wiley & Sons, 2003 (www.the cochranelibrary.com).

6.   Hand C, Harvey I. The effectiveness of topical preparations for the treatment of earwax: a systematic review. *Br J Gen Pract* 2004; 54: 862–867.

Emergency hormonal contraception

An emergency hormonal contraception (EHC) product containing levonorgestrel became available as a Pharmacy medicine in 2001. In 2004, the dosage regimen was changed from two 750 microgram tablets taken 12 hours apart to a single dose of 1500 micrograms. A Cochrane review[1] has confirmed that a single dose of 1500 micrograms of levonorgestrel offers high efficacy as an emergency contraceptive with an acceptable side-effect profile. At the time of reclassification there was considerable debate over the wisdom of making EHC available over the counter; however, recent research[2] appears to confirm that it has not led to an increase in its use, to an increase in unprotected sex, or to a decrease in the use of more reliable methods of contraception.

Active constituent and presentation

Levonelle One Step (Schering Health) is presented as a single tablet containing 1500 micrograms levonorgestrel.

Mode of action and efficacy

Levonorgestrel is thought to act in one of several ways, depending on the point in the menstrual cycle at which it is used.

- Before ovulation it may prevent ovulation by delaying or inhibiting the release of the ovum from the ovary.
- After ovulation it may prevent fertilisation by affecting the motility of the fallopian tube and preventing sperm from meeting the ovum.
- After fertilisation it induces changes in the endometrium that render it unreceptive to the ovum and prevent implantation.

All of the above mechanisms are considered to be contraceptive rather than abortifacient, as, from a clinical viewpoint, fertilisation is not considered to have taken place and a fetus cannot develop until a fertilised ovum is implanted in the endometrium.

Clinical trial data[3] show that, overall, levonorgestrel EHC prevents 85% of expected pregnancies if used within 72 hours of unprotected intercourse, but effectiveness declines with time. It is 95% effective if taken within 24 hours, 85% if used within 24–48 hours, and 58% effective if used within 48–72 hours. It is not licensed for use after 72 hours.

Dosage

Levonorgestrel EHC is licensed for use by women of 16 years and over. The tablet is taken as soon as possible after unprotected sexual intercourse, preferably within 12 hours and not more than 72 hours after. Unprotected intercourse may have occurred because of suspected failure of a barrier method, or if part of a course of an oral contraceptive has been missed. In the latter situation, contraceptive effectiveness can be considered to be compromised, and EHC offered, if intercourse has taken place within 7 days of the following:

- with a combined contraceptive
  - two or more pills missed from the first seven pills in a pack, or
  - four or more pills missed mid-course, or
  - if two or more pills are missed from the last seven in a pack, EHC is not necessary providing that the next pack is started immediately, i.e. without the normal pill-free break.

- with a progestogen-only contraceptive:
  - if one or more pills has been missed or taken more than 3 hours after the usual time.

In all the situations above, additional contraceptive precautions should be taken until consecutive daily pill taking at the correct time has been resumed for at least 7 days.

Taking levonorgestrel EHC may delay or bring forward the onset of the next period by a few days, but should not otherwise disrupt the cycle. Repeated courses are not dangerous, but can disrupt the cycle.

Levonorgestrel EHC is not suitable as a regular means of contraception, and women who ask repeatedly for supplies should be advised to consider long-term methods.

Contraindications

There are very few situations in which levonorgestrel EHC cannot be safely recommended. The only contraindications are:

- hypersensitivity to levonorgestrel
- pregnancy, because it will be ineffective, although there is no evidence that the fetus will be harmed if the preparation is taken by a pregnant woman. (Before making a supply a pharmacist should ask appropriate questions to verify that a prospective purchaser is not already pregnant: if she is pregnant, she should be referred to her doctor)
- severe hepatic dysfunction
- conditions such as severe diarrhoea or Crohn's disease, in which there is a high risk that the medication will not be absorbed.

A relative contraindication is breast cancer, although the risk to a sufferer from the medication is much less than that of pregnancy.

Breastfeeding is not a contraindication as only very small amounts of levonorgestrel appear in breast milk. Any potential problem can be overcome by taking a dose immediately after feeding and not feeding the baby for at least 3 hours after taking a dose.

Side-effects

Side-effects of levonorgestrel EHC are as for progestogens generally and include abdominal pain, headache, dizziness, fatigue and breast tenderness, but these are not usually serious. The main undesirable effect is nausea, which in clinical trials affected 23% of subjects. Vomiting occurred in about 5% of subjects. If vomiting occurs within 3 hours of a dose of levonorgestrel, absorption will be impaired and another dose must be taken as soon as possible. A dose must be kept down for at least 3 hours within 84 hours of intercourse to ensure effectiveness. There are no medications to prevent nausea and vomiting licensed for non-prescription sale in this situation. Antihistamines for motion sickness and domperidone for gastric motility disorders are available without prescription, but supply would be outside of their licensing conditions.

Interactions

Levonorgestrel is metabolised in the liver; drugs which induce liver enzymes will therefore increase its metabolism and could reduce its effectiveness. These drugs include: primidone, phenytoin, carbamazepine, St John's wort, griseofulvin, rifampicin, rifabutin and ritonavir. Levonorgestrel itself inhibits the metabolism of ciclosporin, raising plasma levels and increasing the risk of toxicity. Patients taking any of these drugs should be referred to their doctor.

Other issues

Repeated requests for EHC

Although there is no evidence that repeated use is harmful, levonorgestrel EHC is not intended to be used as a means of regular contraception. Repeated use is also likely to disrupt the menstrual cycle. If a client asks repeatedly for supplies, the pharmacist should explain this and advise on conventional methods of contraception.

Third-party requests for EHC

It is not a requirement of the licensing conditions that the supply of EHC must be made to the client in person. However, a pharmacist is unlikely to be able to obtain all the necessary information from a third party to decide that supply is appropriate. Supply to a third party should therefore be made only in exceptional circumstances.

Requests in advance of need

The licensing conditions for levonorgestrel EHC allow supplies only if unprotected intercourse has occurred within the previous 72 hours, which precludes sales in advance of need. The rationale for this restriction has been questioned by some, who argue that, as an emergency form of contraception, patients should be able to be keep it available for use without delay should the emergency arise.

Age of client

The rate of unplanned teenage pregnancies in the UK is the highest in Europe and, although it has been falling in recent years, there were 8000 conceptions in girls under the age of 16 in 2001, and 3500 abortions. In an attempt to reduce these numbers, several health authorities have introduced schemes allowing pharmacists to supply levonorgestrel EHC to girls under the age of 16 years under patient group directions. However, the licensing conditions for the product do not permit sale for supply to girls under 16 years of age.

Moral objections to supply

Some pharmacists have moral or religious objections to hormonal contraception. Others may be prepared to supply contraceptives but regard EHC as a form of abortion, as they believe that life commences with fertilisation of the ovum and not with implantation of the fertilised ovum into the uterine wall. The Royal Pharmaceutical Society's Code of Ethics respects the rights of such pharmacists not to supply

EHC themselves, but they must not obstruct a client's right to obtain EHC and are expected to treat requests sensitively and advise where a supply can be obtained quickly.

Privacy and confidentiality

It is extremely important that a client is able to discuss a request for EHC with a pharmacist in privacy. Arrangements should be made to facilitate this, and the pharmacist should personally deal with all requests for EHC.

Practice guidance

Full practice guidance for pharmacists on the supply of EHC as a 'pharmacy' medicine is available from the Royal Pharmaceutical Society (http:www.rpsgb.org/members/search/index.html, or by post from the Practice Division).

REFERENCES

1. Cheng L, Gülmezoglu AM, Van Oel CJ, *et al* Interventions for emergency contraception. *The Cochrane Library*, issue 3. Chichester, UK: John Wiley & Sons, 2004 (www.thecochranelibrary.com).
2. Marston C, Meltzer H, Majid A. Impact on contraceptive practice of making emergency hormonal contraception available over the counter in Great Britain: repeated cross sectional surveys. *BMJ* 2005; 331: 271.
3. Ho PC. Emergency contraception: methods and efficacy. *Curr Opin Obstet Gynecol* 2000; 12: 175–179.

Eye conditions

Minor eye conditions for which non-prescription medication is available are: bacterial and allergic conjunctivitis and styes, sore and 'tired' eyes, dry eyes and blepharitis. For preparations for allergic conjunctivitis, see chapter on Hay fever.

Causes and treatment

Bacterial conjunctivitis is an infectious condition affecting one or both eyes, in which the conjunctiva become inflamed. The infecting organism is most often *Staphylococcus aureus*, but several other bacteria may also be responsible. The main symptoms are a feeling of itchiness or grittiness, and there is often also a discharge. There is no pain, and vision is not affected, except for blurring caused by the discharge.

Viruses are also common causative agents of infective conjunctivitis and it may be clinically difficult to distinguish a viral from a bacterial infection. However, over-the-counter treatment of any superficial infective conjunctivitis with an antibacterial agent is considered appropriate, as it may help prevent secondary bacterial infection if the condition is of viral origin.[1]

A stye (external hordeolum) is an infection of the lash follicle of the eyelid, producing pustules. The most common infecting agent is *S. aureus*.

Non-prescription antimicrobial compounds available for the treatment of these infections are:

- chloramphenicol
- propamidine isetionate
- dibromopropamidine isetionate.

Chloramphenicol

Chloramphenicol was reclassified from a Prescription-only medicine to a Pharmacy medicine in 2005. It is an antibiotic originally

developed from strains of *Streptomyces venezuelae* but is now produced synthetically. It is active against a wide range of ocular
pathogens, including *S. aureus*. It is considered the gold standard for
the treatment of conjunctivitis and is the agent against which other
topical treatments are compared.[2]

It penetrates well into the aqueous humour of the eye after
topical application and has low ocular surface toxicity. Development
of resistance is rare.[3,4]

Use and administration

Chloramphenicol eye drops are licensed for use without prescription
for adults and children aged 2 years and over. The dosage is one drop
instilled into the infected eye every 2 hours for the first 48 hours and
4 hourly thereafter, during waking hours only. The course of treatment is 5 days, and should be completed even if symptoms improve.

Side-effects, contraindications and cautions

Side-effects, such as mild stinging or burning in the eye on application
and blurring of vision, are usually minor and transient. Chloramphenicol eye drops should not be used in patients who have a history
of hypersensitivity to chloramphenicol or who have experienced
myelosuppression during previous exposure to chloramphenicol or
those with a family history of blood dyscrasias. The product is not
recommended for pregnant or breastfeeding women. Prolonged or
frequent intermittent topical application of chloramphenicol should
be avoided as it may increase the likelihood of sensitisation and emergence of resistant organisms. The drops should not be used for more
than 5 days, and a doctor should be consulted if symptoms do not
improve within 48 hours of starting treatment. Contact lenses should
not be worn during the course of treatment, and soft contact lenses
should not be replaced for 24 hours after completing the treatment.
In the pharmacy, chloramphenicol eye drops should be stored in a
refrigerator at 2–8°C. Once opened, the drops should be discarded
after 5 days.

Product

- Optrex Infected Eye drops
  Crookes

Propamidine isetionate and dibromopropamidine isetionate

These aromatic diamidine antiseptics are bactericidal against Gram-positive organisms but are less active against Gram-negative bacteria. The first successful treatment of bacterial conjunctivitis with propamidine isetionate was reported in 1944. Since then no clinical research or trials in relation to bacterial eye infections appear to have been published, although there have been some clinical reports on the use of propamidine isetionate in the treatment of acanthamoeba keratitis (a condition beyond the scope of this book). Current clinical opinion is that chloramphenicol is the drug of choice for superficial bacterial eye infections, and the *British National Formulary* regards propamidine and dibromopropamidine as of little value.

Eye drops are formulated with propamidine isetionate 0.1% and eye ointment with dibromopropamidine isetionate 0.15%. Both can be used for adults and children. The ointment persists longer on the corneal surface and needs to be applied only twice daily, but can cause stickiness and blurring of vision. It is suitable for the treatment of both conjunctivitis and styes. The drops need to be used four times daily and are not suitable for styes. Probably the best regimen for conjunctivitis is to use drops during the day and ointment at night. In both conditions, treatment should be continued for 24 hours after symptoms have cleared. If symptoms do not significantly improve within 48 hours, treatment should be discontinued and the patient referred for medical advice.

Cautions

Both formulations may cause slight stinging when applied. Contact lenses should not be worn when either preparation is being used. As with all ophthalmic preparations, products should be discarded not more than 1 month after opening.

Products

As ointment and drops:

- Brolene
  Sanofi-Aventis

- Golden Eye
  Typharm

SORE AND 'TIRED' EYES

Causes and treatment

Redness and mild irritation in the eyes can be caused by activities such as driving and close work, and environmental pollutants. Several products, based mainly on astringents and vasoconstrictors, are available.

Witch hazel

Several products contain distilled witch hazel (hamamelis water), which contains flavonoids and tannins. Witch hazel has astringent and anti-inflammatory properties, but there appears to be no evidence for its efficacy in ophthalmic preparations. Distilled witch hazel is the sole constituent of Optrex Sore Eyes drops (Crookes), and is also a constituent of Optrex Red Eyes drops.

Vasoconstrictor – naphazoline

Mode of action

Naphazoline, a decongestant vasoconstrictor, is included in some ophthalmic preparations to shrink the dilated blood vessels that cause redness. Naphazoline is a sympathomimetic agent with marked alpha-adrenergic activity, with a rapid and prolonged action when applied topically. It is documented as being effective in constricting conjunctival blood vessels, and in reducing discomfort associated with ocular inflammation.[5,6] It is included with distilled witch hazel in Eye Dew and Optrex Red Eyes drops (both Crookes), and is the sole active constituent of Murine (Prestige Brands).

Cautions, contraindications and interactions

Long-term use of decongestant eye drops can lead to rebound congestion (hyperaemia), and a paper has been published documenting a large number of cases of conjunctival inflammation following long-term use.[7] Purchasers should therefore be advised not to use these products continuously. Decongestants may slightly dilate the pupils, so their use should be avoided by patients with glaucoma. Because of the slight risk that these ophthalmic sympathomimetic decongestants may raise blood pressure and interfere with carbohydrate metabolism and thyroid function, patients with high blood pressure, heart disease, diabetes or hyperthyroidism should consult their doctor before using these products.

DRY EYES

Causes and treatment

Dry eye (keratoconjunctivitis sicca), as its name implies, is a chronic condition characterised by dryness of the surface of the eye. It is caused by either a deficiency of conjunctival mucus, due to the absence or significant impairment of the mucin-producing goblet cells of the conjunctiva, or tear deficiency; the latter is often associated with rheumatoid arthritis.

Treatment of dry-eye conditions is usually with tear substitutes ('artificial tears'); several products are available that take slightly different approaches to the problem. The main goal of formulation is to prolong the action of products and reduce the frequency of application required.

The compounds used are:

- hypromellose
- polyvinyl alcohol (PVA)
- carbomer 940
- hydrophobic ocular lubricants.

There is little or no information available on the relative efficacy of tear substitutes. Knowledge of the cause of a patient's dry eye should help with selection of a suitable preparation, but choice is often a matter of patient preference, reached by a process of trial and error.

Hypromellose

Hypromellose (hydroxypropyl methylcellulose) is the only tear-substitute compound available in non-proprietary form. It is a mixed cellulose ether with viscosity-enhancing properties, which prolongs the persistence of the water in the drops, containing it on the surface of the eye. It is most useful for dry eyes caused by tear deficiency (e.g. Sjögren's syndrome associated with rheumatoid arthritis). Viscosity of hypromellose solutions increases with concentration, and it has been suggested that the 0.3% concentration of the official formulation may be too low.[8] On the other hand, too high a concentration can lead to blurring and crusting. The optimum range appears to be 0.5–1%. Dextran 70 0.1% is included with hypromellose 0.3% in Tears Naturale (Alcon) as a fluid volume expander. pH also seems to be an important factor in relation to the comfort of the drops in the eye, slightly alkaline formulations being thought preferable; the official preparation has a pH of 8.5.

Products

- Hypromellose Eye Drops BP (0.3%)
- Isopto Alkaline (1%)
- Isopto Plain (0.5%)
- Tears Naturale (0.3%)
  all *Alcon*

Polyvinyl alcohol (PVA)

PVA is a viscosity enhancer, usually used at a concentration of 1.4%. It also promotes wetting of the ocular surface, and is useful to help spread the water content of the drops over the eye when the mucus layer is deficient and tear film distribution is patchy. Like hypromellose, PVA enhances stability of the tear film without causing ocular irritation or toxicity. Liquifilm Tears Preservative-Free (Allergan) and Refresh (Allergan) also contain povidone, which is thought to mimic the action of natural conjunctival mucin.

Products

The following contain PVA 1.4%

- Liquifilm Tears
- Liquifilm Tears Preservative-Free
- Refresh Ophthalmic (single-use vials)
  all *Allergan*

- SnoTears
  Bausch & Lomb

Carbomer 940

This is an acrylic acid polymer that is formulated as a liquid gel for the treatment of dry eye. Its claimed advantages include ease of application and prolonged contact with the corneal surface, requiring application only three or four times a day. In one trial, a carbomer 940 gel-based product was found to remain on the cornea for seven times longer than a conventional PVA-based formulation.[9]

Products

- GelTears
  Bausch & Lomb

- Viscotears liquid gel
  Novartis Ophthalmics

Hydrophobic ocular lubricants

These are sterilised ointments containing liquid and soft paraffins and wool fat or a similar non-lanolin derivative. They mimic the lipid layer of human tear film and are intended mainly for night-time use to protect and lubricate the cornea during sleep.

Products
- Simple Eye Ointment (non-proprietary)
- Lacri-lube
  Allergan

- Lubri-Tears
  Alcon

BLEPHARITIS

Blepharitis is inflammation of the margins of the eyelids, often accompanied by crusting. In many cases the cause is unknown, but it is sometimes associated with seborrhoea of the scalp. In these cases, treatment of the scalp with an antidandruff shampoo containing pyrithione zinc, selenium sulphide or ketoconazole may resolve the condition (see chapter on Dandruff and seborrhoeic dermatitis). The hydrophobic ocular lubricants discussed above can be used to soften crusts.

ADMINISTRATION OF EYE DROPS AND OINTMENT

The following technique is recommended for the most effective use of eye drops and ointment.

- Wash hands thoroughly.
- Tilt head backwards.
- Gently grasp lower outer eyelid just below the lashes and pull the eyelid away from the eye.

- Place the dropper or ointment tube directly over the eye by looking directly at it.
- With drops:
  - just before applying a drop, look upwards
  - after applying a single drop, look downward for several seconds
  - release the eyelid slowly
  - keep eyes closed for 1–2 minutes
  - with a finger, gently press over the opening of the tear duct in the inner corner of the eye
  - blot excess liquid from around the eye.

- With ointment:
  - with a sweeping motion, insert 1–2 cm ointment inside the lower lid
  - release the eyelid slowly
  - keep eyes closed for 1–2 minutes
  - blot excess ointment from around the eye.

PRODUCT SELECTION POINTS

- Chloramphenicol is now the treatment of choice for bacterial conjunctivitis. Propamidine and dibromopropamidine isetionates have been used with apparent safety and effectiveness for many years, although without supporting clinical evidence. However, bacterial conjunctivitis is a self-limiting condition that is likely to resolve within a few days without treatment, and doubt has been cast on whether there is any need for antibiotic treatment.[10]
- Dibromopropamidine isetionate is the only non-prescription antibacterial compound licensed for the treatment of styes.
- Naphazoline appears to be an effective ocular decongestant for the treatment of sore and 'tired' eyes resulting from trivial causes, but prolonged, continuous use should be avoided.

- Several tear-substitute products, based on three main active constituents, are available for the treatment of dry eye conditions. Choice is often a matter of patient preference.

PRODUCT RECOMMENDATIONS

- For bacterial conjunctivitis – chloramphenicol eye drops.
- For styes – dibromopropamidine isetionate eye ointment.
- For sore and 'tired' eyes resulting from mild ocular congestion – eye drops containing naphazoline.
- For dry eye conditions – choice often dependent on patient preference.

REFERENCES

1. Royal Pharmaceutical Society. *Practice guidance: OTC chloramphenicol eye drops.* London: Royal Pharmaceutical Society, 2005.
2. Titcomb LC. Topical ocular antibiotics: part 1. *Pharm J* 2000; 264: 298–301.
3. Seal DV, Barrett SP, McGill JI. Aetiology and treatment of acute bacterial infection of the external eye. *Br J Ophthalmol* 1982; 66: 357–360.
4. Beasley H, Boltralik JJ, Baldwin HA. Chloramphenicol in aqueous humour after topical application. *Arch Ophthalmol* 1975; 93: 184–185.
5. Swedish GP Allergy Team. Topical levocabastine compared with oral loratadine for the treatment of seasonal allergic rhinoconjunctivitis. *Allergy* 1994; 49: 611–615.
6. Abelson MB, Paradis A, George MA, *et al.* Effects of Vasocon-A in the allergen challenge model of acute allergic conjunctivitis. *Arch Ophthalmol* 1990; 108: 520–524.
7. Soparkar CN, Wilhelmus KR, Koch DD, *et al.* Acute and chronic conjunctivitis due to over-the-counter ophthalmic decongestants. *Arch Ophthalmol* 1997; 115: 34–38.
8. Toda I, Shinozaki N, Tsubota K. Hydroxypropyl methylcellulose for the treatment of severe dry eye associated with Sjogren's syndrome. *Cornea* 1996; 15: 120–128.
9. Leibowitz HM, Chang RK, Mandell AI. Gel tears. A new medication for the treatment of dry eyes. *Ophthalmology* 1984; 91: 1199–1204.
10. Rose PW, Harnden A, Brueggemann AB, *et al.* Chloramphenicol treatment for acute infective conjunctivitis in children in primary care: a randomised double-blind placebo-controlled trial. *Lancet* 2005; 366: 37–43.

FURTHER READING

For a further account of non-prescription treatments for minor eye conditions see: Titcomb LC. Over-the-counter ophthalmic preparations. *Pharm J* 2000; 264: 212–218.

Fungal nail infection (onychomycosis)

Onychomycosis is a fungal infection of the nail plate of the fingers or toes. Infection of the toenails accounts for 80% of cases. The main infecting organisms are dermatophytes (principally *Trichophyton rubrum*), when the condition is known as tinea unguium, and this accounts for 85–90% of infections. However, infection can also be caused by various yeasts and moulds. It is quite a common condition, with a prevalence of 3–8%. Incidence has been increasing with a growing use of communal areas such as swimming pools and showers and wearing of occlusive footwear. The most common clinical form of the condition is distal subungual onychomycosis, characterised by onycholysis (separation of the nail plate from the nail bed), and the nail becomes discoloured (white, yellow or brown) and thickened or brittle.

TREATMENT

Amorolfine 5% nail lacquer

Mode of action, efficacy and safety

Amorolfine nail lacquer was reclassified from POM to P status in 2006. Amorolfine is a morpholine derivative which is used topically as an antifungal agent. It has a broad spectrum of activity, including dermatophytes, other fungi and yeasts. Its fungicidal action is based on an alteration of the fungal cell membrane targeted primarily on sterol biosynthesis, resulting in depletion of ergosterol and accumulation of ignosterol in fungal cytoplasmic membrane, causing the fungal cell wall to thicken and chitin deposits to form inside and outside the cell wall. The nail lacquer formulation builds a non-water soluble film on the nail plate which remains at the application site for 1 week and acts as a depot for the drug. Continuous use for a minimum of 6 months is usually required to eradicate infections. A randomised clinical trial[1] involving 456 patients had an overall cure rate of 46% with overall improvement in a further 24% of patients after weekly treatment for six months with amorolfine 5% nail lacquer. Almost no adverse effects were reported. The manufacturers report[2] an incidence of about 1 in 200 000 minor adverse reactions, mainly a slight burning sensation and irritation. Amorolfine is not systematically absorbed and there are no interactions with other drugs.

Licensing conditions and use

Amorolfine 5% nail lacquer is licensed for treatment of mild cases of the most common and easily recognised types – distal and lateral – of onychomycosis, affecting up to two nails, in adults from 18 years of age. It is not licensed for sale in pregnancy or if breastfeeding, or if a patient has any underlying conditions predisposing to fungal nail infections, such as peripheral circulatory disorders, diabetes mellitus or if the patient is immunocompromised or immunosuppressed. It should not be supplied if there is nail dystrophy or the nail plate is destroyed.

The lacquer should be applied once weekly. The pack size is 3 ml, sufficient for about 3 months' treatment, after which treatment and progress of the condition should be reviewed. Treatment should be continued until the infected section of nail has completely grown out, which takes about 6 months for fingernails and 9–12 months for toenails. Detailed directions for use, together with materials for applying the lacquer, are supplied with the product.

Product

- Curanail Lacquer
  Galderma

Monphytol paint (LAB)

This preparation is a rapidly-drying non-greasy paint, containing meythyl and propyl undecenoates, salicylic acid and chlorobutanol. It is licensed as a P medicine for the treatment of athlete's foot, tinea unguium and other fungal infections of the skin. Undecenoates are effective in mild chronic cases of tinea pedis.[3] Salicylic acid is a

keratolytic agent that promotes the removal of the infected keratinised tissue of skin and nails. Chlorobutanol has antibacterial and
antifungal properties. Monphytol paint must be applied at least twice
daily. A systematic review[4] found insufficient evidence to draw con-
clusions on the effectiveness of topical treatments for fungal nail
infections.

REFERENCES

1.   Reinel D. Topical treatment of onychomycosis with amorolfine 5% nail
      lacquer: comparative efficacy and tolerability of once and twice weekly use.
      Dermatology 1992; 184 (Suppl 1): 21–24.
2.   Medicines and Healthcare products Regulatory Agency. Consultation
      Document: ARM 31. Request to reclassify a product from POM to P:
      Curanail Lacquer. (www.mhra.gov.uk/home/idcplg?IdcService=SS_GET_
      PAGE&nodeId=433&within=Yes&keywords=amorolfine) (Accessed 27
      January 2006).
3.   Chretien JH, Esswein JG, Sharpe LM, *et al.* Efficacy of undecylenic acid-
      zinc undecylenate powder in culture positive tinea pedis. *Int J Dermatol*
      1980; 19: 51–54.
4.   Crawford F, Hart R, Bell-Syer S, *et al.* Topical treatments for fungal infec-
      tions of the skin and nails of the foot. *Cochrane Database Syst Rev* 2000;
      (1): CD001434.

Haemorrhoids

Haemorrhoids ('piles') are estimated to affect at least 50% of the adult population at some time. Incidence is equal in both sexes and is highest in individuals between 20 and 50 years of age. Embarrassment over the site of the lesion and the need for a rectal examination may deter some patients from seeking medical attention as early as they might for other conditions. It is therefore important for pharmacists to have a sound knowledge of the symptoms and to know when patients should be advised to see a doctor.

CAUSES

Haemorrhoids are the result of swelling and dilatation of the veins that line the anal canal. They are classified into two types: internal haemorrhoids, which are confined to the anal canal and are not visible, and external haemorrhoids, which become enlarged through straining at defecation and prolapse through the anal sphincter to protrude outside the anus. External piles either retract spontaneously after defecation or can be pushed back inside by the patient with a finger; if straining at defecation is not addressed and corrected, the haemorrhoids may remain prolapsed.

Symptoms of haemorrhoids include pain and discomfort, as a result of swelling in the area of the rectum and anus, which often becomes worse on defecation. Itching and a burning sensation also occur. Pruritus ani is intense itching around the anus which is often associated with haemorrhoids. It may result, in part, from irritation caused by seepage of rectal contents because of sphincter dysfunction.

Internal piles may bleed. The blood will be fresh and bright red in colour and may be seen on the faeces and splashed around the toilet bowel after defecation. Although this is not normally serious, any patient with rectal bleeding should be referred.

Haemorrhoids are often self-diagnosed and mild cases can be treated without medical intervention, although recurrent episodes or those that fail to clear up within a week should be referred.

TREATMENT

Most cases of haemorrhoids can be managed by local symptomatic treatment, together with use of laxatives where necessary (see chapter on Constipation). Dietary adjustment is also an important contributory factor, as constipation is often caused by a low-residue diet.

A wide range of products, in a variety of dosage forms, for the symptomatic treatment of haemorrhoids is available without prescription (see table on page 178). Most products contain a combination of ingredients. The rationale for the use of most of these seems logical but, as is often the case with non-prescription medicines, there is little objective evidence of their effectiveness. The various types of ingredients are reviewed below.

Local anaesthetics

Compounds available

Compounds available are:

- benzocaine
- cinchocaine
- lidocaine.

Mode of action, uses and adverse effects

Local anaesthetics reversibly block excitation of pain receptors and sensory nerve fibres in and around the area of application. Local anaesthetics used in haemorrhoidal preparations are weak basic amines with the same basic chemical structure of an aromatic lipophilic group joined to a hydrophilic amino group by a linking ester or amide moiety. They reach their site of action by penetrating the lipophilic nerve structure in their lipid-soluble uncharged form, but exert their anaesthetic action in the ionised form. All compounds used in haemorrhoidal preparations, except for benzocaine, are

Haemorrhoidal products and constituents

Constituent type	Constituent	Product	Manufacturer	Dosage form
Local anaesthetic	Benzocaine	Lanacane	Coombe	C
	Cinchocaine	Nupercainal	LPC	O
	Lidocaine	Anodesyn	Thornton & Ross	O, S
		Germoloids	Bayer	C, O, S
		Hemocane	LPC	C
Astringents	Allantoin	Anodesyn	Thornton & Ross	O, S
	Bismuth oxide	Anusol	Pfizer Consumer Healthcare	C, O, S
		Anusol Plus HC		O, S
	Hamamelis (witch hazel)	Preparation H Clear Gel	Wyeth	G
	Peru balsam	Anusol	Wyeth	C, O, S
		Anusol Plus HC	Wyeth	O, S
	Zinc oxide	Anusol	Wyeth	C, O, S
		Anusol Plus HC	Wyeth	O, S
		Germoloids	Wyeth	C, O, S
		Hemocane	Wyeth	C
Anti-inflammatory	Hydrocortisone	Anusol Plus HC	Wyeth	O, S
		Germoloids HC	Wyeth	Sp
		Perinal	Wyeth	Sp
Fibrinolytic	Mucopolysaccharide polysulphate	Anacal	Sankyo	O, S
Sclerosing agent	Lauromacrogol	Anacal	Sankyo	O, S
Skin protectant	Shark liver oil	Preparation H	Sankyo	O, S
Wound-healing agent	Yeast cell extract	Preparation H	Sankyo	O, S

C, cream; G, gel; O, ointment; S, suppository; Sp, aerosol spray.

hydrochloride salts which are converted to the base at tissue pH. Benzocaine is used in the free base form.

At the cellular level, the ionised form of the anaesthetic blocks conduction of nerve impulses across cell membranes by decreasing their permeability to cations, mainly sodium ions. The degree of penetration and effectiveness of individual compounds depend on their lipid solubility, dissociation constants and on the pH of the surrounding environment, which is often influenced by the formulation of the product. Compounds with high lipid solubility tend to be more potent and have a faster onset and longer duration of action than those with low lipid solubility. (Local anaesthetics are less effective on inflamed than on normal tissue as the pH of inflamed tissue is lower, resulting in a higher degree of ionisation, leaving less of the uncharged lipophilic drug available to penetrate the tissues.) Generally, amide-type anaesthetics are more potent and produce less sensitisation than ester-type compounds.

Local anaesthetics are included in haemorrhoidal preparations to relieve pain, burning and itching. Use should be restricted to the perianal region and lower anal canal; local anaesthetics should not be used in the rectum as there is little sensory tissue there and anaesthetic can be rapidly absorbed through the rectal mucosa to cause potentially toxic systemic effects. Local anaesthetics are also absorbed rapidly through damaged skin. Skin sensitisation and systemic allergic reactions are possible with prolonged use, and use should be restricted to 5–7 days.

Benzocaine is an ester-type local anaesthetic. Allergic reactions and sensitisation have been reported relatively frequently. Recommended concentrations are in the range 5–10%, with a frequency of application of up to six times daily. Lanacane cream (Combe International), which is licensed for the treatment of anal irritation, contains 3% benzocaine, which would appear too low a concentration to be effective; the recommended application is three times daily. The concentration may be deliberately low in order to reduce the possibility of sensitivity reactions.

Cinchocaine is a potent and long-acting amide-type compound, included at concentrations of 0.5–1% in haemorrhoidal preparations. It has less sensitising potential than benzocaine.

Lidocaine is an amide-type compound with a relatively long duration of action and is the local anaesthetic most widely used in haemorrhoidal preparations. Although it is poorly absorbed through the skin, lidocaine may be rapidly and almost completely absorbed through mucous membranes and broken skin, and can cause systemic toxicity. However, most non-prescription formulations contain low concentrations and are safe if used in accordance with the manufacturer's directions.

Astringents

Compounds available

Compounds available are:

- allantoin
- bismuth oxide
- bismuth subgallate
- witch hazel (hamamelis) extract
- Peru balsam
- zinc oxide.

Mode of action and uses

Astringents coagulate protein in skin and mucous membrane cells to form a superficial protective layer. By reducing the secretion of mucus and intracellular contents from damaged cells, they help relieve local irritation and inflammation. Some astringent substances, such as zinc oxide and bismuth salts, also provide a mechanical protective barrier on the surface of damaged skin; Peru balsam has additional mild antiseptic properties.

The US licensing authorities have suggested that, in products containing constituents with a mechanical protective effect, astringents should constitute at least 50% of the dosage unit, in order to provide a protective layer of adequate thickness. This level is not reached in any of the products marketed in the UK, however.

Anti-inflammatories

Compound available

There is only one compound – hydrocortisone acetate.

Mode of action and uses

Hydrocortisone has a long history of prescription usage as a topical anti-inflammatory. (For a description of the mechanism of action of hydrocortisone, see the chapter on Mouth ulcers.) Haemorrhoidal preparations containing hydrocortisone have been available on prescription for many years. Hydrocortisone was reclassified from a Prescription-only medicine to a Pharmacy medicine in 1987 for limited dermatological indications, and in 1995 licensing was extended for use in haemorrhoidal preparations.

Products available

Three brands are available:

- Anusol Plus HC ointment and suppositories (containing 0.25% hydrocortisone acetate in the ointment and 10 mg per suppository, together with astringent constituents)
  Pfizer Consumer Healthcare

- Germoloids HC spray (containing 0.2% hydrocortisone with 1% lidocaine hydrochloride)
  Bayer

- Perinal spray (containing 0.2% hydrocortisone with 1% lidocaine hydrochloride)
  Dermal

Use of haemorrhoidal preparations containing hydrocortisone is subject to several licensing restrictions: they should not be used for patients under 18 years of age, or during pregnancy or breastfeeding. They should not be used for more than 7 days.

The possibility of infection should be excluded before starting use because of the possibility of immunosuppression by the corticosteroid. The manufacturer of Anusol Plus HC advises that the product should not be recommended to new sufferers who have not consulted their doctor, and that its use should be reserved for the relief of pain associated with the inflammation of more severe haemorrhoids.

Other agents

Fibrinolytic agent

Mucopolysaccharide polysulphate has a chemical structure similar to that of heparin. It is claimed to promote fibrinolysis and to break up small blood clots, and also to possess anti-inflammatory and anti-exudative properties. It is also claimed to strengthen weak connective tissue in the anus and rectum. There is little evidence of its effectiveness, although a trial found that a paste consisting of a proteolytic enzyme and heparin significantly improved the healing and resolution of acutely inflamed haemorrhoids.[1]

Sclerosing agent

Lauromacrogol 400 is a non-ionic surfactant that has been used as a sclerosing agent in the treatment of varicose veins. Sclerotherapy involves injecting a sclerosing agent into a varicosed vein to create fibrosis and close off the lumen; the technique is used, although rarely, for the treatment of haemorrhoids. There appears to be no evidence that lauromacrogol 400 is effective when applied externally.

Skin protectant

Shark liver oil has been used as a source of vitamin A, and both it and cod liver oil have been used as skin protectants. However, claims of their value have not been substantiated by controlled observations, and a US Food and Drug Administration advisory review panel found a lack of demonstrated effectiveness for both substances.

Wound-healing agent

Yeast cell extract is a water-soluble extract of brewer's yeast, claimed to be effective in promoting wound healing and tissue repair in haemorrhoids. Extensive tests have been carried out in *in vitro* and *in vivo* wound-healing models, and the substance has been found to stimulate oxygen consumption, increase angiogenesis and promote collagen synthesis; however, no acceptable evidence exists that it has any effect on haemorrhoids.

Administration and dosage forms

The recommended treatment regimen for most preparations is twice daily, morning and evening, and after each bowel movement; products containing hydrocortisone should not be used more than three or four times in 24 hours. The bases of all products are likely to contribute an additional emollient and soothing effect, and the lubricating effect of suppositories may ease straining at stool. However, suppositories may slip into the rectum and melt there, bypassing the anal areas where the medication is needed and increasing the possibility of systemic absorption of local anaesthetics and hydrocortisone. This possibility is increased if the patient is lying down. Creams and ointments are generally considered to be preferable to suppositories for self-treatment of haemorrhoids.

PRODUCT SELECTION POINTS

- There is little evidence for the effectiveness of non-prescription haemorrhoidal preparations, but most have been available and used with apparent satisfaction for many years, and some are also prescribed frequently. The bases of products may themselves have a soothing effect.
- Products containing a local anaesthetic and constituents with mechanical protective or astringent properties would appear to be logical choices, as long as the content of these is sufficient to exert an effect.

- Products containing hydrocortisone may be useful for inflammation and irritation associated with haemorrhoids and pruritus ani, and may also be worth trying if other products have not proved effective.
- Creams and ointments are considered preferable to suppositories.

PRODUCT RECOMMENDATIONS

- For mild cases – a compound preparation containing a local anaesthetic and astringent or skin-protective constituents.
- For cases with additional inflammation and irritation – a preparation containing hydrocortisone.
- For underlying constipation – short-term treatment with a stimulant laxative, followed by an increase in fibre and fluid in the diet or regular use of a bulk laxative.

REFERENCE

1.   Gupta PJ. Use of enzyme and heparin paste in acute haemorrhoids. *Rom J Gastroenterol* 2002; 11: 191–195.

Hay fever

(continued . . .)

Hay fever (seasonal allergic rhinitis) affects as many as 12% of the population and the incidence is thought to be increasing. However, it appears that only about 20% of sufferers consult their doctor, and this is now perhaps less necessary because most treatments for hay fever have become available without prescription as a result of reclassification from Prescription-only medicines to Pharmacy medicines.

Non-prescription treatments for hay fever are available in both oral and topical formulations. Ingredients in oral products include antihistamines (both sedative and non-sedative) and combinations of sedative antihistamines with decongestants. Topical formulations include products for use in the nose and in the eyes.

CAUSES

Hay fever is the result of a type I allergic reaction, in which initial exposure of a sensitive individual to an antigen (usually tree or grass pollens) results in the production of antigen-specific immunoglobulin E (IgE). IgE attaches to mast cells and basophils, which become sensitive to further antigenic material. On further exposure, the antigen binds to IgE, causing degranulation of the mast cells and release of chemical mediators (including histamine), leukotrienes and prostaglandins, which produce the inflammatory response. Prolonged exposure to the allergen may result in sustained response, causing nasal congestion.

TREATMENT – ORAL FORMULATIONS

Histamine is the principal chemical mediator responsible for the inflammatory response of hay fever (and other allergic reactions). All oral formulations for treatment of hay fever are antihistamines and act as competitive antagonists at the H_1-receptor.

The older, sedative antihistamines (known as first-generation antihistamines) are lipophilic and cross the blood–brain barrier readily. In the brain, in addition to binding to H_1-receptors, sedative antihistamines bind to and block muscarinic (cholinergic) receptors and, in some cases, alpha-adrenoceptors and serotonergic receptors. As a result, they cause several generally undesirable side-effects such as sedation, dry mouth, blurred vision, urinary retention, constipation and gastrointestinal disturbances.

The newer non-sedative antihistamines (second-generation antihistamines) are less lipophilic and do not penetrate the brain to a significant extent; they are therefore much less likely to cause centrally mediated side-effects. However, about 6% of individuals exhibit drowsiness and other central side-effects in response to placebo; in addition, impairment of function, if it occurs, is not always accompanied by subjective feelings of drowsiness. Patients should therefore be warned that these antihistamines may affect driving and other skilled tasks, and that excess alcohol intake should be avoided.

Antihistamines are generally effective in controlling the symptoms of hay fever, including sneezing, nasal itching, rhinorrhoea and, to a lesser extent, allergic conjunctivitis, but have little or no effect on nasal congestion. The maximum effect of antihistamines is not achieved until several hours after peak serum levels have been reached; in addition they cannot reverse the consequences of H_1-receptor activation, and are effective only if they are able to block histamine release before it occurs. For maximum effectiveness, therefore, antihistamines should be taken when symptoms are expected, rather than after they have started.

Non-sedative antihistamines

Compounds available

Compounds available are:

- acrivastine
- cetirizine
- loratadine.

Uses

These compounds are used mainly for the treatment of hay fever and perennial rhinitis, but they are also licensed for the treatment of insect bites and allergic skin reactions. However, because of their lack of central activity they are of no use for motion sickness. In hay fever, they are generally preferable to the older antihistamines because of the much lower incidence of side-effects, but they are slightly more expensive. All drugs in this group are of equal efficacy.[1] Acrivastine has a rapid onset of action and a short half-life, necessitating more frequent dosing than cetirizine or loratadine, but it may be useful to give rapid relief. Peak plasma levels of cetirizine and loratadine are reached in about 1 hour; they have a long elimination half-life and are long acting, requiring only once-daily dosage. Loratadine is metabolised in the liver by cytochrome P450 isoenzymes CYP3A4 and CYP2D6, and theoretically can interact with drugs that inhibit or are metabolised by these enzymes. Interactions have been demonstrated experimentally, and the manufacturer advises that plasma concentrations may be increased by ketoconazole.

The incidence of sedation is extremely low for all three drugs[2] (fewer than one patient in 140 complained of drowsiness with any of these drugs in a prescription-event monitoring study of more than 43 000 patients). Loratadine is associated with a much lower incidence of sedation than acrivastine or cetirizine, and has been recommended as the antihistamine of choice for people in occupations in which any degree of sedation is undesirable.[2]

Dosage

- **Acrivastine:** adults and children over 12 years, 8 mg three times daily (not recommended for use in children under 12 years or people over 65 years).
- **Cetirizine:** adults and children over 12 years, 10 mg daily (not licensed for children under 12 years).
- **Loratadine:** adults and children over 6 years, 10 mg daily.

Product examples

All products are Pharmacy medicines unless indicated otherwise.

- Acrivastine
  — Benadryl Allergy Relief capsules (in Benadryl Plus Capsules acrivastine is formulated with a sympathomimetic decongestant [pseudoephedrine])
    Pfizer Consumer Healthcare

- Cetirizine
  — AllerTek tablets (GSL)
    Ratiopharm
  — Benadryl Allergy Oral Solution
  — Benadryl One A day Allergy Relief tablets (GSL)
    both *Pfizer Consumer Healthcare*
  — Piriteze Allergy syrup (GSL) and tablets
    GSK Consumer Healthcare
  — Zirtek Allergy tablets
    UCB Pharma
  — Zirtek Allergy Relief tablets (GSL)
  — Zirtek Allergy solution
  — Zirtek Allergy Relief for Children (GSL)

- Loratadine
  — Clarityn Allergy tablets and syrup
    Schering-Plough (tablets, 7 pack GSL)

Sedative antihistamines

Compounds available

Compounds available are:

- chlorphenamine
- clemastine
- diphenhydramine
- promethazine.

Uses

There is no evidence of difference in effectiveness between older anti-histamines, although individual response to specific drugs varies widely. Choice is often based on personal preference and factors such as degree of sedation caused and duration of action, which do differ between compounds. Price may also be a factor.

Promethazine is highly sedative but has a long half-life, and a single dose may provide relief of symptoms for up to 24 hours. The dose is preferably taken at night, on the supposition that the sedative effect will have largely worn off by the following morning. Clemastine has an intermediate sedative effect (about 20% greater than placebo) and a duration of action of up to 12 hours. Chlorphenamine is about as sedating as clemastine, with a faster onset but shorter duration of action; it is also the cheapest oral antihistamine. Diphenhydramine has pronounced sedative properties.

Dosage

- **Chlorphenamine:** adults and children over 12 years, 4 mg 3–4 times daily; children 6–12 years, 2 mg.
- **Clemastine:** adults and children over 12 years, 1 mg twice daily; children 6–12 years, 0.5 mg.

- **Diphenhydramine:** adults and children over 12 years, 75–200 mg daily (not recommended for children under 12 years).
- **Promethazine:** adults and children over 12 years, 25–50 mg at night, or 10–20 mg two or three times daily; children over 5 years, 10–25 mg daily.

Side-effects, cautions and interactions

See above, and the chapter on Cough.

Product examples

- Chlorphenamine
    - Hayleve
      Chatfield Laboratories
    - Piriton Allergy tablets and syrup
      GSK Consumer Healthcare
    - Pollenase Antihistamine tablets and syrup
      Peach Ethical

- Clemastine
    - Tavegil elixir and tablets
      Novartis Consumer Health

- Diphenhydramine
    - Histergan syrup and tablets
      Norma Chemicals

- Promethazine
    - Phenergan elixir and tablets
      Sanofi-Aventis

Combination products

Some oral products that contain combinations of antihistamines with sympathomimetic decongestants are marketed for treating nasal congestion associated with hay fever and the common cold. (See also chapter on Colds; for a description of systemic sympathomimetic decongestant compounds, see chapter on Cough.) Antihistamines on their own are effective for treating the typical symptoms of acute hay fever, known as the early phase. Prolongation of the condition by continued exposure to the allergen leads to a late-phase sustained response, producing mucus secretion in the nasal passages and increased permeability of the capillaries, resulting in submucosal swelling and blockage. First-generation antihistamines reduce rhinorrhoea through their antimuscarinic action but do little to relieve nasal congestion, but co-administration of a sympathomimetic decongestant may be helpful. Several trials have found antihistamine–decongestant combinations to be more effective than an antihistamine alone.[3–5]

Combination products marketed for hay fever include:

- Benadryl Plus capsules (acrivastine/pseudoephedrine)
  Pfizer Consumer Healthcare

- Haymine tablets (chlorphenamine/ephedrine)
  Forest

- Multi-action Actifed syrup and tablets (triprolidine/ pseudoephedrine)
  Pfizer Consumer Healthcare

TREATMENT – NASAL PREPARATIONS

Nasal preparations contain anti-inflammatory, sympathomimetic decongestant or antihistamine constituents.

Anti-inflammatory agents

Compounds available

Compounds available are:

- beclometasone
- fluticasone
- sodium cromoglicate.

Budesonide and flunisolide are classified as Pharmacy medicines, although currently no over-the-counter products are available.

Mode of action

Beclometasone and fluticasone are corticosteroids. They down-regulate the inflammatory response of type I allergic reactions by reducing the number of basophils and mast cells and blocking release of mediator substances. They inhibit both early and late responses to allergen exposure, and are therefore effective in relieving nasal congestion. Intranasal corticosteroids are now regarded as the treatment of choice for moderate-to-severe hay fever and are superior to oral antihistamines.[6]

Sodium cromoglicate is known as a mast-cell stabiliser, although its mode of action is not entirely understood. Mast-cell stabilisers were originally thought to act by stabilising mast-cell membranes and preventing their degranulation, but new evidence indicates that other factors are involved. They are effective against both early and late type I responses.

Uses and dosage

Beclometasone, fluticasone and sodium cromoglicate are used intranasally. (Sodium cromoglicate can also be used in the eyes; see below.) As they counteract both the early and late response to allergen exposure, they are effective in relieving all nasal symptoms of hay fever, including congestion. They take some days to achieve optimum effect, and treatment should ideally be started at least 2 weeks before symptoms are expected.

Beclometasone and fluticasone

Beclometasone and fluticasone are presented as aqueous non-aerosol sprays, because pressurised sprays are thought to be more likely to cause local reactions. Absorption from the nasal mucosa is low, and systemic effects are highly unlikely at recommended doses; any local reactions, such as stinging, burning and aftertaste, are mild and transient. Both drugs have been found to be effective and safe in use; there is some evidence that fluticasone may be superior and faster acting.[7,8]

Patients should be advised that if symptoms are already present when treatment is started then it may be several days before an effect is noted and several weeks before full relief is obtained. Long-term use appears to be safe. Treatment may need to be maintained throughout the hay fever season, and repeated each year. The recommended adult dosage is two sprays twice a day.

Beclometasone and fluticasone are licensed for use in adults of 18 years and over. They should be avoided if there is infection in the nose or eye. Pregnant and breastfeeding women should seek medical advice before use. There are otherwise no significant contraindications or interactions.

Sodium cromoglicate

Sodium cromoglicate is available as an aqueous spray containing 4% sodium cromoglicate (Rynacrom [Pantheon Healthcare]). Sodium cromoglicate is a prophylactic agent; treatment should therefore be initiated before the pollen season starts and continued throughout. It is less effective at controlling nasal symptoms than corticosteroids, and has the disadvantage of requiring administration at least four times daily. However, it is very safe and is suitable for children from 5 years of age. There are no specific cautions or contraindications associated with its use, and it does not interact with other drugs.

Products

- Beclometasone

  — Beconase Hayfever spray
    GSK Consumer Healthcare

  — Beconase Hayfever Relief for Adults nasal spray
    GSK Consumer Healthcare

  — Care Hay fever spray
    Thornton & Ross

  — Vivabec spray
    Lexon UK

- Fluticasone

  — Flixonase Allergy nasal spray
    GSK Consumer Healthcare

- Sodium cromoglicate

  — Rynacrom 4% nasal spray
    Pantheon Healthcare

Antihistamines

Compound available

The following compound is available:

- azelastine.

Azelastine

Azelastine is a second-generation antihistamine. It is a potent long-acting anti-allergic compound with marked H_1-antagonist properties. It is marketed in the UK without prescription for intranasal and ocular use, and has only local activity at the doses administered. It has been found to be as effective as oral loratadine and cetirizine in controlling the symptoms of rhinitis, but with varying results when compared with intranasal corticosteroids.[9] Twice-daily use is recommended.

Intranasal azelastine is not licensed for over-the-counter sale for use in children under 5 years, and caution is recommended for use in pregnant and breastfeeding women. The maximum recommended treatment period without medical supervision is 1 month.

Product

- Azelastine
  — Aller-eze nasal spray
    Novartis Consumer Health

Sympathomimetic decongestants

Drops and sprays containing sympathomimetic decongestants are used to relieve nasal congestion associated with hay fever, and may be useful to begin treatment when the nose is badly blocked. (For further details, see the chapter on Colds.)

TREATMENT – EYE PREPARATIONS

Compounds available

The following compounds are available:

- sodium cromoglicate
- lodoxamide
- antihistamine/sympathomimetic decongestant combinations.

Sodium cromoglicate

Most eye symptoms relating to hay fever will be controlled by oral antihistamines; however, if symptoms are persistent or particularly troublesome, sodium cromoglicate 2% eye drops are usually effective.[10] Several proprietary brands are available. Sodium cromoglicate is particularly useful if hay fever symptoms occur only in the eyes, where it exerts an action rapidly.[11] It is used four times daily, and can be used in children.

Lodoxamide

Lodoxamide is a mast-cell stabiliser. It is licensed for the treatment of seasonal conjunctivitis in adults and children of 4 years and over, administered four times daily.

In clinical trials,[12,13] lodoxamide has been found to be equivalent or superior to sodium cromoglicate in the treatment of allergic conjunctivitis.

Antihistamine/decongestant combination

Otrivine-Antistin eye drops (Novartis Consumer Health) contain an antihistamine, antazoline sulphate 0.5%, and xylometazoline hydrochloride 0.05%. The latter ingredient has vasoconstrictor action and is included as a conjunctival decongestant. This preparation can be used for the short-term treatment of hay fever symptoms; however, prolonged use may raise intraocular pressure and precipitate glaucoma. The drops are used twice or three times daily and are suitable for use in children from 5 years of age.

Products

- Sodium cromoglicate
  - Clarityn Allergy eye drops
    Schering-Plough
  - Opticrom Allergy eye drops
    Sanofi-Aventis
  - Optrex Allergy eye drops
    Crookes
  - Pollenase Allergy eye drops
    Peach Ethical

— Vivicrom eye drops
  Nucare

- Lodoxamide

  — Alomide Allergy eye drops
    Alcon

- Antihistamine/decongestant

  — Otrivine-Antistin eye drops
    Novartis Consumer Health

Caution for contact lens wearers

All eye drop preparations for allergic conjunctivitis contain benzalkonium chloride as preservative. This is absorbed into soft contact lenses and released on to the cornea during wear, causing inflammation and irritation. Contact lenses should not be worn while using these products.

PRODUCT SELECTION POINTS

- Oral antihistamines are the first-line treatment for mild or occasional hay fever, and are usually effective against all acute (early-phase) symptoms. Treatment is more effective if commenced when symptoms are expected rather than after they have started.
- All antihistamines, both first- and second-generation, are more or less equally effective, although response can vary between individuals.
- Second-generation antihistamines are usually the first choice for recommendation, given the low risk of sedation and anticholinergic side-effects. Of these, loratadine has the least potential for sedation.

- The degree of sedation caused by first-generation antihistamines varies between compounds; some cause relatively little, and some patients do not experience drowsiness at all. In addition, as first-generation antihistamines are generally cheaper than second-generation compounds, the former are often a suitable choice.
- First-generation antihistamines are generally best avoided in elderly patients, given their anticholinergic side-effects and the need to avoid use in patients with glaucoma or prostatic hypertrophy. In any case, hay fever is unusual in the elderly and patients with symptoms of this condition should be referred to their GP.
- Beclometasone or fluticasone nasal spray, plus a second-generation antihistamine if necessary, are the first choice for more persistent symptoms and nasal congestion. Oral combination products containing first-generation antihistamines and sympathomimetics are not the treatment of choice, because of side-effects, cautions and contraindications associated with both classes of drugs, and because they should not be used long term.
- Beclometasone and fluticasone are more effective for treating severe or persistent nasal symptoms of hay fever than sodium cromoglicate, but use is confined to individuals over 18 years of age. Sodium cromoglicate can be used in children from the age of 5 years and is licensed for use in pregnancy. Both are safe to use throughout the hay fever season. Azelastine is also effective, and can be used in children from the age of 12 years.
- Sodium cromoglicate eye drops provide fast and effective relief for eye symptoms associated with hay fever, and are safe to use for prolonged periods. Lodoxamide appears to be at least as effective.

PRODUCT RECOMMENDATIONS

- Oral antihistamines
  - Loratadine or cetirizine: second-generation, non-sedative, no reported interactions or side-effects, once-daily dosing
  - Chlorphenamine: first-generation, relatively little sedation, cheapest oral antihistamine
  - Loratadine: for children from 2 years of age, non-sedating

- Nasal products (severe nasal symptoms and congestion)
  - Adults: azelastine may be more effective for sneezing, itchy eyes, itchy nose, and watery eyes, while beclometasone or fluticasone are more effective for the relief of nasal congestion
  - Children: Rynacrom Allergy nasal spray

- Eye drops
  - For severe eye symptoms: sodium cromoglicate and lodoxamide are both effective.

REFERENCES

1. Slater JW, Zechnich AD, Haxby DG. Second-generation antihistamines: a comparative review. *Drugs* 1999; 57: 31–47.
2. Mann RD, Pearce GL, Dunn N, Shakir S. Sedation with 'non-sedating' antihistamines: four prescription-event monitoring studies in general practice. *BMJ* 2000; 320: 1184–1186.
3. Pleskow W, Grubbe R, Weiss S, Lutsky B. Efficacy and safety of an extended-release formulation of desloratadine and pseudoephedrine vs the individual components in the treatment of seasonal allergic rhinitis. *Ann Allergy Asthma Immunol* 2005; 94: 348–354.
4. Sussman GL, Mason J, Compton D, *et al*. The efficacy and safety of fexofenadine HCl and pseudoephedrine, alone and in combination, in seasonal allergic rhinitis. *J Allergy Clin Immunol* 1999; 104: 100–106.
5. Nuutinen J, Holopainen E, Malmberg H, *et al*. Terfenadine with or without phenylpropanolamine in the treatment of seasonal allergic rhinitis. *Clin Exp Allergy* 1989; 19: 603–608.

6. National Prescribing Centre. Common questions about hay fever. *MeReC Bulletin* 2004; 14, Number 5.
7.   LaForce CF, Dockhorn RJ, Findlay SR, *et al.* Fluticasone propionate: an effective alternative treatment for seasonal allergic rhinitis in adults and adolescents. *J Fam Pract* 1994; 38: 145–152.
8. van As A, Bronsky EA, Dockhorn RJ, *et al.* Once daily fluticasone propionate is as effective for perennial allergic rhinitis as twice daily beclomethasone diproprionate. *J Allergy Clin Immunol* 1993; 91: 1146–1154.
9. Golden SJ, Craig TJ. Efficacy and safety of azelastine nasal spray for the treatment of allergic rhinitis. *J Am Osteopath Assoc* 1999; 99 (7 Suppl): S7–S12.
10. Lindsay-Miller AC. Group comparative trial of 2% sodium cromoglycate (Opticrom) with placebo in the treatment of seasonal allergic conjunctivitis. *Clin Allergy* 1979; 9: 271–275.
11. Montan P, Zetterstrom O, Eliasson E, Stromquist LH. Topical sodium cromoglycate (Opticrom) relieves ongoing symptoms of allergic conjunctivitis within 2 minutes. *Allergy* 1994; 49: 637–640.
12. Verin P, Allewaert R, Joyaux JC, *et al.*; Lodoxamide Study Group. Comparison of lodoxamide 0.1% ophthalmic solution and levocabastine 0.05% ophthalmic suspension in vernal keratoconjunctivitis. *Eur J Ophthalmol* 2001; 11: 120–125.
13. Avunduk AM, Avunduk MC, Kapicioglu Z, *et al.* Mechanisms and comparison of anti-allergic efficacy of topical lodoxamide and cromolyn sodium treatment in vernal keratoconjunctivitis. *Ophthalmology* 2000; 107: 1333–1337.

Head lice

CAUSE

Head lice are small wingless insects (*Pediculus humanus capitis*) that live on and suck blood from the scalp. Infestation may remain unnoticed for several weeks until an allergic response to lice saliva begins to cause intense itching, or perhaps until parents are alerted to an epidemic at their child's school.

The female louse lays a daily batch of tiny pale eggs (nits), attached to the hairs close to the scalp. Adult lice may live for up to several weeks. Infection is spread by direct head-to-head contact, and possibly by transfer through contact with infected hairbrushes, hats, pillows etc., although lice cannot survive for long away from the scalp.

The condition is most common in children aged 4–11 years and is more common in girls than boys; anybody can be infected, however. The length or state of cleanliness of the hair makes little difference to the likelihood of becoming infected.

TREATMENT

Several insecticides (pediculocides) are available for the eradication of head lice, in presentations including aqueous and alcoholic lotions, a shampoo, a creme rinse and a mousse. All are licensed as Pharmacy medicines. Some of these preparations are also licensed for the treatment of crab lice and scabies (see chapter on Scabies). Products containing carbaryl were also Pharmacy medicines until 1995, when they were reclassified as Prescription-only medicines because it was found that carbaryl was carcinogenic when fed to laboratory animals at high doses over long periods. A non-insecticidal treatment containing 4% dimeticone became available in 2006.

Head lice can also be removed by a mechanical method – wet combing or 'bug busting' – without the use of any chemical-based preparations, and a head-lice repellent, piperonal, is also available.

Insecticides

The insecticides (pediculocides) available without prescription for the treatment of head lice are:

- malathion
- permethrin
- phenothrin.

Malathion

Mode of action

Also known as carbofos, malathion is an organophosphorus compound. It is a potent cholinesterase inhibitor, preventing the breakdown of acetylcholine and interfering with neuromuscular transmission in the head louse, paralysing it and preventing it from feeding. Malathion is oil soluble and is absorbed by a process of passive diffusion through the lipid coat of both insect and egg; achieving a lethal dose depends on the concentration of the product and the duration of contact. Ovicidal activity of all pediculocides is increased by the incorporation of an alcohol into the preparation base; alcohol-based insecticides are also less likely to produce resistance.[1] Malathion is poorly absorbed through human skin, and it is also much more efficiently detoxified by human metabolic processes than by those of insects. It is therefore safe for occasional or intermittent use at low concentrations as a pediculocide.

Administration

Aqueous solutions are rubbed gently into the scalp until all the hair and scalp is thoroughly moistened; application should extend to the neck area and behind the ears. Treatment failure often occurs because the insecticide does not reach all of the scalp. The hair should be allowed to dry naturally, as malathion is inactivated by heat. The solution is left on for 12 hours, usually overnight, and the hair is then shampooed in the normal way. The hair should be combed with a fine-toothed comb while it is still wet, to remove dead and dying lice from the scalp and empty egg cases attached to the hair shafts. A second application after 7 days is recommended to kill any lice emerging from eggs that may have survived the initial treatment.

Alcoholic lotions are applied in the same way as aqueous lotions. It is important that heat is not applied to dry the hair, given the flammable nature of the vehicle. The room should be well ventilated, with no naked flames or lighted objects.

The *British National Formulary* states that the shampoo is much less effective than lotions because, although it is more concentrated, it is diluted 15–30 times with water when applied, it has a much shorter time in contact with the hair and scalp, and the insecticide may be inactivated by hot water. To apply, the hair should be thoroughly wetted and sufficient shampoo applied to work up a rich lather and cover the entire scalp and neck area. The shampoo is left on for at least 5 minutes, rinsed off and the process repeated. The hair is then wet combed, as described above. The procedure must be carried out three times at 3-day intervals. Shampoo formulations of pediculocides have been shown to be much less effective than lotions.[2]

Contraindications, cautions and side-effects

There are no contraindications to the use of malathion, apart from known sensitivity. Preparations are not contraindicated in pregnant or breastfeeding women, although manufacturers recommend caution. Alcoholic lotions should not be used for asthmatic patients and young children, as the isopropyl alcohol in the vehicle may precipitate bronchospasm. Nor should they be used for patients with eczema, as alcohol may cause inflammation and stinging.

All preparations may affect permed, coloured or bleached hair. The only reported side-effect of malathion preparations is very rare skin irritation.

Products

- Aqueous lotions (0.5%)
  - Derbac-M liquid
    SSL International

- Quellada M liquid
  GSK Consumer Healthcare

- Alcoholic lotions (0.5% in isopropyl alcohol)
  - Prioderm lotion
  - Suleo-M lotion
    both *SSL International*

- Shampoo (1%)
  - Prioderm shampoo
    SSL International

All the above are licensed for use in patients aged from 6 months.

Permethrin and phenothrin

Mode of action

Natural pyrethrum, extracted from pyrethrum flowers (*Chrysanthemum cinerariaefolium, Compositae*), has been used as a horticultural pesticide for many years. Pyrethrins are effective insecticides with low mammalian toxicity, but the naturally occurring compounds are unstable when exposed to light. Photostable synthetic pyrethroids have been developed in recent years, and the first pyrethroid pediculocide product was introduced in the UK in 1990. Pyrethroids are rapidly absorbed across the insect cuticle and exert their action on the sodium channels of louse nerve axons, causing initial excitement and then paralysis.

Administration

Phenothrin is available as an alcoholic lotion and an aqueous liquid, used in the same way as malathion alcoholic lotions and liquids, and as a mousse, which is left on the hair for 30 minutes and then washed off using an ordinary shampoo. Permethrin creme rinse is applied after the final rinse after using an ordinary shampoo. The hair is towel-dried, and creme rinse is applied in sufficient quantity to coat the scalp and hair fully. The preparation is rinsed off after 10 minutes and the hair wet combed.

Contraindications, cautions and side-effects

The manufacturers recommend that Lyclear is avoided in pregnancy and during breastfeeding.

Products

- Permethrin

  — Lyclear Creme Rinse (1% in a creme rinse base with 20% isopropyl alcohol)
  Warner Lambert

- Phenothrin

  — Full Marks lotion (0.2% in an alcoholic base)
  — Full Marks liquid (0.2% in an aqueous base)
  — Full Marks mousse (0.5%)
  all *SSL International*

Dimeticone

Dimeticone lotion does not have conventional insecticide activity. It contains 4% long-chain linear silicone (dimeticone) in a volatile silicone base (cyclomethicone). It is applied in the same way as other lotions for head-lice infestation. It appears to act against head lice by coating the insects and thus disrupting their ability to manage water.[3]

Product

- Hedrin lotion
  Thornton & Ross

Wet combing ('Bug busting')

Wet combing has been recommended as an alternative method for tackling the problem of head lice and resistance without the use of insecticides. The technique involves combing wet hair with a fine-tooth comb for about 30 minutes after shampooing and using conditioner. If evidence of lice is found, the process should be repeated twice weekly for 2 weeks to remove lice emerging from eggs before they can spread.

Piperonal

Mode of action

Piperonal is presented as an aqueous–alcoholic solution in a pump spray. It has a sweet floral odour resembling heliotrope and occurs naturally in the oils of some plants; it is widely used in foods and perfumery. Its mechanism of action is unknown, but it is thought to provoke a negative response from the lice antennae receptors, causing them to avoid movement into treated areas.

Piperonal has been shown to be effective in the laboratory 'Arena' test, which is designed to compare repellent effects of different materials.[4] The test is performed by placing the same number of lice on two filter-paper discs; half of one of the discs is treated with the test substance. Lice move around in a completely random manner, and under normal conditions after a given time, would be expected to be evenly distributed on the discs. The test showed a 93% inhibition of lice on the half-disc treated with piperonal compared with the control disc. Piperonal has no insecticidal activity.

Administration

The product should only be used on heads that are clear of infestation. It is sprayed onto the hair once daily during periods when infection is likely. The normal precautions should be employed with people who are asthmatic or have a sensitive skin, and use is not recommended for children under 2 years of age; otherwise there are no restrictions. The main use of the product is to prevent inadvertent re-infestation after treatment with insecticides, before all cases have been traced and the lice eradicated. It is not intended to be used as a routine prophylactic.

Product

- Rappell
  Chefaro UK

Efficacy and resistance

A Cochrane systematic review[5] has concluded that permethrin, pyrethrin and malathion are effective in the treatment of head lice, although the quality of trials reviewed was very poor and only four of 71 studies met the inclusion criteria. In the single trial conducted so far,[3] dimeticone lotion was found to be about equivalent in efficacy to phenothrin but to be less irritant.

Evidence for the effectiveness of wet combing is conflicting. The largest trial so far [6] (over 4000 patients) led to the conclusion that it was much less successful than malathion in eradicating infection and that it should not be regarded as a first-line treatment. However, a smaller more recent trial[7] found that it was four times more effective than chemical products for eliminating head lice.

Over the last 15–20 years, head lice have developed resistance to commonly used pediculocides through natural selection, making it increasingly difficult to eliminate infestations, and there is no direct contemporary evidence of the comparative effectiveness of the available pediculocides. Choice is probably best made on the basis of local resistance patterns. Little resistance appears to have developed to carbaryl, which seems to justify its remaining as a Prescription-only medicine of last resort.[8]

Rotational policies to limit the development of resistance, whereby health authorities recommended a specific pediculocide to be used exclusively in an area for a period of usually 3 years, followed by other compounds in rotation for 3 years each, have now been abandoned and replaced by the mosaic method of treatment. Here, no particular pediculocide is recommended, but as patients come forward for treatment they are each given a different pediculocide in rotation.

Two applications of insecticide 1 week apart is now recommended as standard treatment. If one compound fails to effect a cure, a different one should be used for the next treatment.

Resistance to pediculocides is also encouraged by people, usually worried parents, trying to prevent re-infestation by using them, particularly shampoos, as prophylaxis, in the mistaken belief that routine use of these in place of ordinary shampoos will keep the family clear of lice. Another misconception is that if one family member is infested the entire family should be treated. However, there is no point in trying to eradicate lice unless their presence is confirmed, and unnecessary treatment merely contributes towards the possibility of resistance. Lice are almost always passed on from one person to another by head-to-head contact. The way to eradicate infestations and prevent recurrences is by tracing and checking everybody with whom an infested person is likely to have had such close contact over the preceding few weeks, and to treat all those found to be infested.

Apparent treatment failure with pediculocides is quite frequent, and is often suggested to be because of the ineffectiveness of the products. The more likely cause, however, is either incorrect use of products or rapid re-infestation following successful treatment.[9] Contact tracing to prevent re-infestation, as described above, is therefore extremely important.

PRODUCT SELECTION POINTS

- There is no clear evidence that any one pediculocide is significantly more effective than the others. All should be effective if used correctly.

- Alcoholic lotions may be more effective than aqueous lotions, but are not suitable for patients with asthma or eczema, or in young children.
- Two applications of pediculocide 1 week apart is now recommended as standard treatment.
- A mosaic policy should be used for selection of pediculocide.
- Shampoos are much less effective than lotions and are not recommended.
- Head-lice products should not be used for prophylaxis, as they are usually not effective and their use in this way encourages the development of resistance. Tracing infested contacts and eliminating lice from them is the most effective way to prevent re-infestation.
- Piperonal spray can be used as a lice repellent to prevent re-infestation during outbreaks while contacts are being traced. It is not intended for routine prophylactic use.
- Wet combing ('bug busting') is an alternative method for identifying and eliminating head lice without the use of insecticides, but requires heavy commitment; its efficacy is uncertain.

PRODUCT RECOMMENDATIONS

In the absence of contraindications, an alcohol-based malathion or pyrethroid preparation is recommended as first choice.

REFERENCES

1.   Burgess I. Concern over the development of resistance to pyrethroid head lice treatments. *Pharm J* 1995; 255: 490.
2.   Armoni M, Bibi H, Schlesinger M, *et al*. Pediculosis capitis: why prefer a solution to shampoo or spray? *Pediatr Dermatol* 1988; 5: 273–275.
3.   Burgess IF, Brown CM, Lee PN. Treatment of head louse infestation with 4% dimeticone lotion: randomised controlled equivalence trial. *BMJ* 2005; 330: 1423–1426.
4.   Peock S, Maunder JW. Arena tests with piperonal, a new louse repellent. *J R Soc Health* 1993; 113: 292–294.

5.   Dodd CS. Interventions for treating headlice. *The Cochrane Library*, issue 2. Chichester, UK: John Wiley & Sons, 2001 (www.thecochrane library.com).

6.   Roberts RJ, Casey D, Morgan DA, Petrovic M. Comparison of wet combing with malathion for treatment of head lice in the UK: a pragmatic randomised controlled trial. *Lancet* 2000; 356: 540–544.

7.   Hill N, Moor G, Cameron MM, *et al*. Single blind randomised controlled trial comparing the Bug Buster kit with over the counter insecticide treatments against head lice in the United Kingdom. *BMJ* 2005; 331: 384–387.

8.   Downs AM, Stafford KA, Hunt LP, *et al*. Widespread insecticide resistance in head lice to the over-the-counter pediculocides in England, and the emergence of carbaryl resistance. *Br J Dermatol* 2002; 146: 88–93.

9.   Meinking TL. Clinical update on resistance and treatment of *Pediculosis capitis*. *Am J Manag Care* 2004; 10 (9 Suppl): S264–S268.

Indigestion

(continued . . .)

Indigestion and dyspepsia are terms commonly used interchangeably to describe a range of somewhat vague symptoms in the upper gastrointestinal tract that are generally associated with the ingestion of food.

There are several possible causative factors, but whatever the cause, moderately raising stomach pH generally relieves symptoms. Treatment is therefore aimed at either neutralising gastric acid or suppressing its secretion.

Antacids have traditionally been the main form of treatment, and some compounds additionally form a protective layer over the gastric mucosa. Indigestion medicines often contain ingredients to control associated symptoms such as wind, gastric reflux and colicky spasm. As with other categories of self-medication, indigestion remedies often contain more than one constituent. H_2-receptor antagonists and a proton pump inhibitor, which reduce gastric acid production, are also available as over-the-counter treatments.

TREATMENT - ANTACIDS

Mode of action

Several alkali metal salts are used in the treatment of indigestion. These are weak bases which dissociate to form alkaline salts, thereby neutralising gastric acid. Antacids used in indigestion treatments have differing neutralising capacities, and the degree to which they are absorbed systemically also varies, influencing their duration of action. Soluble salts act quickly but are absorbed rapidly, so reducing their duration of action, while salts of divalent and trivalent metal ions are insoluble and have a less rapid but more prolonged action. The ideal antacid would be fast acting, with a high neutralising capacity, not absorbed into the body, and with a long duration of action. No single compound possesses all these attributes, but combinations are formulated in an attempt to produce medicines with most of the benefits and a minimum of drawbacks. This means that antacid medicines are usually combinations of two or more compounds, each contributing to the neutralising capacity of the product. The amount of each compound is therefore less than would be required to achieve neutralisation on its own.

Compounds used

The compounds used as antacids are:

- sodium and potassium bicarbonates
- calcium carbonate
- aluminium hydroxide
- magnesium and bismuth salts
- magnesium–aluminium complexes.

These compounds, together with their actions, uses, dosage, side-effects and cautions, are considered individually below. Given the huge number of antacid products available, examples are given for each antacid compound rather than at the end of the section. Interactions for all antacids are discussed as a separate topic at the end of the section.

Sodium bicarbonate

Action, uses and dosage

This compound has been a traditional household standby for the treatment of indigestion because it is cheap, fast acting and effective. It is also a standard ingredient in formulary preparations such as Magnesium Trisilicate Mixture BP, Magnesium Trisilicate Tablets, Compound, BP and Aromatic Magnesium Carbonate Mixture BP.

Carbon dioxide is generated during neutralisation of acid with sodium bicarbonate, and excess gas escapes through eructation (belching). This helps to relieve the distension of the stomach that can contribute to the discomfort of dyspepsia. The antacid dose of sodium bicarbonate is 1–5 g.

Side-effects and cautions

The main disadvantage of sodium bicarbonate is that it is highly soluble and is absorbed systemically; prolonged use can therefore lead to sodium overload and alkalosis. Excess sodium intake can lead to water retention, causing an increase in blood pressure and load on the heart. Products containing significant amounts of sodium bicarbonate are therefore best avoided by patients with hypertension, cardiovascular or renal disease, those on a salt-restricted diet and also in pregnancy. In these individuals, while the occasional dose is unlikely to be harmful, regular use may cause problems. Many antacids that contain either no sodium or insignificant amounts (less than 1 mmol sodium or 85 mg sodium bicarbonate per dose) are available. Regular use of sodium bicarbonate may also cause 'acid rebound' in which there is an increase in stomach acid production. The *British National Formulary* considers that sodium bicarbonate should no longer be prescribed for the relief of dyspepsia.

Potassium bicarbonate

Potassium bicarbonate is used as an alternative to sodium bicarbonate. Hyperkalaemia is possible with prolonged regular use in patients taking potassium-sparing diuretics or angiotensin-converting enzyme inhibitors; otherwise, there are no specific contraindications.

Potassium bicarbonate is included in two indigestion remedy brands, one of which, Algicon tablets (Sanofi-Aventis), has a high sugar content, which should be taken into account if recommending this product to a patient with diabetes.

Product examples

- Algicon suspension and tablets
  Sanofi-Aventis

- Gaviscon Advance Suspension
  Reckitt Benckiser

Calcium carbonate

Action, uses and dosage

Calcium carbonate has the greatest neutralising capacity of all antacids; it is also cheap and long acting. It is a popular ingredient in proprietary products, both alone and in combination with other antacids. The antacid dose range is between 500 mg and 1 g.

Side-effects and cautions

Although calcium carbonate is safe in normal use, problems may arise with excessive usage. The calcium chloride formed during neutralisation of stomach acid is soluble and partially absorbed and can cause hypercalcaemia. Long-term use, especially if large quantities of milk and sodium bicarbonate (perhaps as an antacid ingredient) are also ingested, can give rise to a condition known as milk alkali syndrome, causing nausea, headache and possibly renal damage. Calcium carbonate is also associated with acid rebound, and can cause constipation. Regular use of antacids containing calcium carbonate should be avoided by patients taking thiazide diuretics, as these reduce calcium excretion and hypercalcaemia may result.

Product examples

Containing calcium carbonate as sole antacid constituent

- Remegel tablets
  SSL International

- Rennie Rap-eze tablets
- Rennie Soft Chews
  both *Bayer*

- Setlers antacid tablets
  Thornton & Ross

- Tums tablets
  GSK Consumer Healthcare

Calcium carbonate combined with other antacids

- Bisodol indigestion relief tablets and powder
  Forest

- Rennie Deflatine
- Rennie Liquid Relief
  both *Bayer*

Aluminium hydroxide

Action, uses and dosage

Aluminium hydroxide reacts with gastric acid to form an insoluble colloid, which is not absorbed to a significant extent and is effective for much longer than a rapidly absorbed soluble salt. It also lines the gastric mucosa and acts as a mechanical barrier against excess acid. As an antacid, aluminium hydroxide is given in doses of up to 1 g.

Side-effects and cautions

Aluminium hydroxide is rarely used alone in antacid preparations for several reasons. Used on its own, it can bind to phosphate in the gastrointestinal tract, forming an insoluble complex which, over a long period, may interfere with phosphate and bone metabolism. This can give rise to bone and central nervous system problems, particularly in patients with renal disease. Products containing aluminium hydroxide as sole constituent are used to treat indigestion, but by virtue of their phosphate-binding action they are also used to treat hyperphosphataemia.

In recent years, a correlation has been shown between aluminium in water and Alzheimer's disease, but so far no link has been demonstrated with aluminium-containing antacids. Aluminium hydroxide also tends to cause constipation, but this is often overcome by formulating it with a magnesium salt, which has the opposite effect (see below).

The adsorptive capacity of aluminium hydroxide and its persistence in the gastrointestinal tract can retard the absorption of vitamins and some drugs, including tetracyclines (see Interactions below).

Product examples

Containing aluminium hydroxide as sole constituent

- Aluminium Hydroxide Mixture and Aluminium Hydroxide Tablets

- Alu-Cap capsules
  3M

Magnesium salts

Action and uses

The magnesium compounds used in antacid preparations are the trisilicate, hydroxide, oxide and carbonate. They possess similar properties to aluminium hydroxide, and in addition they tend to increase the tone of the gastro–oesophageal sphincter, useful in treating gastric reflux.

Side-effects and cautions

Magnesium salts are absorbed to a greater extent than aluminium salts, and excessive use, particularly in the presence of renal insufficiency, may lead to hypermagnesaemia, with serious cardiovascular and neurological consequences. Magnesium salts are osmotic laxatives and some compounds are licensed for this use (e.g. magnesium hydroxide in Phillips Milk of Magnesia Liquid [GSK Consumer Healthcare]). In general, however, diarrhoea is an undesirable side-effect in antacids, and is overcome by co-formulating magnesium salts with aluminium hydroxide. The dose of each component is lower than in sole-ingredient products, which minimises the possibility of adverse effects through absorption.

Magnesium trisilicate, found in Magnesium Trisilicate Mixture BP, was once the most popular of formulary antacids but is now little favoured. It is slower acting and has less neutralising capacity than other magnesium salts. It has been reported to cause renal stones because of its silica content, and may also cause other renal damage with chronic use.

Product examples

Containing magnesium hydroxide as sole constituent

- Bisodol indigestion relief powder and tablets
  Forest

- Phillips Milk of Magnesia liquid and tablets
  GSK Consumer Healthcare

Magnesium salts in combination

- Aromatic Magnesium Carbonate Mixture BP
- Maalox Suspension
  Sanofi-Aventis

- Valonorm powder
  Zenith

Bismuth salts

Actions and uses

Bismuth salts have similar properties to aluminium and magnesium salts, neutralising acid and coating the gastric mucosa, thus protecting it against acid attack.

Side-effects and cautions

Long-term use may lead to absorption and neurological damage. Salicylate is absorbed following the administration of bismuth salicylate and may cause the same adverse effects as aspirin. The same precautions should therefore be applied to Pepto-Bismol (bismuth salicylate) as for aspirin, and it should be avoided by aspirin-sensitive individuals and in pregnancy. Bismuth salicylate may be converted to bismuth sulphide in the gut, causing blackening of the faeces and tongue.

Product example

- Pepto-Bismol (bismuth salicylate) suspension and tablets
  Procter & Gamble

Aluminium–magnesium complexes

Aluminium and magnesium compounds have been combined in various ways in an attempt to achieve faster acid neutralisation, longer action and lower absorption. These include:

- magaldrate (aluminium magnesium hydroxide sulphate), contained in Bisodol Heartburn Relief Tablets (Forest)
- hydrotalcite (aluminium magnesium carbonate hydroxide hydrate; claimed to maintain buffering in the optimum pH range for over 2 hours), contained in Altacite Plus Suspension (Peckforton)
- aluminium hydroxide/magnesium carbonate co-dried gel (a co-precipitate of these two compounds, dried to contain a proportion of water for antacid activity), contained in Algicon suspension and tablets (Sanofi-Aventis)
- alexitol (a sodium hydroxyaluminium carbonate–hexitol complex), contained in Actal Tablets (Merck Consumer Health).

There appears to be little evidence to demonstrate an advantage for these products over straightforward aluminium–magnesium salt combinations.

Interactions

Antacids can interfere with the absorption of many drugs. They inter-act with tetracyclines, quinolone antibacterials (e.g. ciprofloxacin, norfloxacin and ofloxacin) and penicillamine to form insoluble metal ion chelates. The absorption of tetracyclines and the antifungals, keto-conazole and itraconazole, is reduced in the presence of antacids as these drugs are less readily soluble in an alkaline than in acid medium. Other commonly prescribed drugs whose absorption is likely to be reduced in the presence of antacids include azithromycin, nitrofuran-toin, rifampicin, phenytoin, chloroquine, phenothiazine anti-psychotics and bisphosphonates.

Antacids also interact with enteric-coated tablets, capsules and granules. These products are formulated to resist gastric acid and dis-solve in the more alkaline medium of the duodenum, releasing the drug there. Enteric coatings may be disrupted prematurely in the pres-ence of antacids, causing unwanted release of the drug in the stomach. Because antacids can interfere with the absorption of so many drugs, patients might be best advised to leave an interval of at least 2 hours between taking a dose of an antacid and any other medicine.

Antacid preparations containing sodium bicarbonate should be avoided by patients on lithium therapy. Sodium ions are preferentially reabsorbed in the kidney, increasing lithium excretion and reducing plasma lithium concentrations.

Formulation and dosage

Liquids and powders generally provide faster relief and have greater neutralising capacity than tablets, as they are very quickly mixed with the stomach contents and their small particle size provides a large contact surface area for neutralising activity.

Advantages of tablets over liquids include ease of portability and administration, and claims have been made for more prolonged action in some cases. Patients generally prefer tablets to liquids.

Tablets should not be swallowed whole, but should be chewed to initiate disintegration or sucked to provide a relatively slow but sustained delivery of antacid to the stomach. The tabletting process can also influence the speed of action. Older formulary preparations, such as Magnesium Trisilicate Compound Tablets BP, may disintegrate relatively slow, but most proprietary tablets are formulated to optimise disintegration and availability. Some novel formulations have been developed to improve both speed of action and palatability.

Timing of the dose also influences the effectiveness of antacids. Antacids should not be taken before or immediately after meals, as peristalsis stimulated by the presence of food accelerates transit and reduces the length of contact of the antacid with the stomach contents. It has been shown that antacids exert the most prolonged effect when taken 1 hour after meals.[1]

Antacid tablet formulations may contain large amounts of sugar in order to make them palatable, which should be considered when making recommendations to patients with diabetes.

Additional ingredients – alginates

Alginates used as additional ingredients with antacids are:

- alginic acid
- magnesium alginate
- sodium alginate

Mode of action

Alginates act as reflux suppressants. Reflux of acidic stomach contents into the oesophagus is normally prevented by the lower oesophageal sphincter (LOS) at the junction of the oesophagus and stomach, which acts as a non-return valve. Several factors can contribute to reducing the muscle tone of the LOS, allowing gastric contents back into the oesophagus. These include certain foods and drinks, alcohol, smoking, some drugs, obesity, pregnancy and anatomical abnormality. Unlike the stomach lining, the oesophageal mucosa has no protection against gastric acid and an irritant process ensues, giving rise to the characteristic symptoms of reflux oesophagitis – 'heartburn' and 'waterbrash'. Reflux oesophagitis is also known as gastric reflux, or simply reflux.

Alginates precipitate out in the acidic medium of the stomach to form a sponge-like polymer matrix of alginic acid. Carbon dioxide bubbles, generated by the reaction between stomach acid and the sodium or potassium bicarbonate included in alginate-containing preparations, become trapped in the matrix and make it buoyant so that it floats on top of the stomach contents like a raft, hence the name 'rafting agents' by which alginate-containing products are sometimes known. When peristalsis occurs, the stomach contents are pushed up against the diaphragm and the alginate raft, which is claimed to form a physical barrier against the reflux of stomach contents into the oesophagus, is forced towards the gastro–oesophageal junction. Aluminium and magnesium antacid salts are included in reflux-suppressant formulations because they help to neutralise stomach contents and any material that is refluxed through the LOS. Gastric alkalinisation is also thought to improve sphincter tone.

Alginate-antacid preparations appear to be more effective than antacids alone in the treatment of reflux oesophagitis, but less so than H_2-antagonists or proton pump inhibitors, although they act more quickly.[2–4]

Products

- Alginic acid
  - Bisodol Heartburn Relief Tablets
    Forest
  - Gastrocote tablets
    Thornton & Ross
  - Gaviscon 250 and Gaviscon Extra Strength Tablets
    Reckitt Benckiser

- — Topal tablets
  Ceuta

- • Magnesium alginate
  - — Algicon suspension
    Sanofi-Aventis

- • Sodium alginate
  - — Acidex suspension
    Pinewood
  - — Gastrocote liquid
    Thornton & Ross
  - — Gaviscon liquid
  - — Gaviscon Advance suspension
  - — Gaviscon Cool Tablets
    all *Reckitt Benckiser*
  - — Rennie DUO suspension
    Bayer

Additional ingredients – antiflatulents and carminatives

Compounds used as additional ingredients with antacids are:

- • simeticone (activated dimeticone)
- • peppermint oil
- • aromatic cardamom tincture
- • capsicum tincture.

Mode of action

Distension of the stomach caused by trapped gas often contributes to the discomfort of indigestion. Simeticone is a silicone-derivative surface-active agent. Its surfactant activity helps to coalesce small gas bubbles into larger ones, which are then vented by eructation.

Peppermint and other volatile oils also have antifoaming (surfactant) properties; they are used for this action and for the warming sensation that they produce in the stomach through mild local counterirritation. However, volatile oils are also smooth muscle relaxants and may aggravate gastric reflux by relaxing the LOS.

Volatile oils and silicones have been shown to be effective in relieving gaseousness, but there is no clear evidence that they are more effective than antacids alone.[5,6]

Product examples

- Simeticone
  — Actonorm gel
    Wallace
  — Altacite Plus suspension
    Peckforton
  — Asilone Antacid liquid and tablets
  — Asilone suspension
    both *Thornton & Ross*
  — Bisodol Wind Relief Tablets
    Forest
  — Kolanticon gel
    Peckforton
  — Maalox Plus suspension and tablets
    Sanofi-Aventis
  — Remegel Wind Relief chewable tablets
    SSL International
  — Rennie Deflatine tablets
    Bayer
  — Wind-Eze tablets
    GSK Consumer Healthcare

All the above products contain antacid compounds, except Wind-Eze tablets, which contain only simeticone.

Aromatic Tincture of Cardamom BP is a constituent of Aromatic Magnesium Carbonate Mixture BP, and this and capsicum tincture are contained in Jackson's Indian Brandee (Herbal Concepts). Peppermint oil is used as a flavouring in many indigestion remedies.

Additional ingredients – antispasmodics

Antispasmodic compounds used as additional ingredients with antacids are:

- atropine
- dicycloverine (dicyclomine).

Mode of action

Colicky spasm is sometimes a feature of dyspepsia, and antimuscarinic drugs are used in some indigestion remedies for their antispasmodic properties. These drugs exert a relaxant effect on gastrointestinal smooth muscle and inhibit gastric secretion through competitive inhibition of acetylcholine at postganglionic parasympathetic effector sites. Antispasmodics are either naturally occurring alkaloids derived from solanaceous herbs or chemically related synthetic compounds.

Antispasmodics used in indigestion remedies fall into two groups: tertiary amines, which are relatively lipid soluble and cross the blood–brain barrier readily, and quaternary ammonium compounds, which are less lipid soluble and less are likely to be absorbed or to cross the blood–brain barrier. The tertiary amines are therefore more likely to produce the undesirable centrally mediated side-effects associated with antimuscarinic drugs, namely dry mouth, blurring of vision, urinary retention, constipation and confusion. The quaternary ammonium compounds may, however, still produce some side-effects, though less pronounced, through direct peripheral activity. Since they are smooth muscle relaxants, antimuscarinic antispasmodics may exacerbate gastric reflux.

Dicycloverine hydrochloride is a tertiary amine, with weaker anticholinergic activity than atropine but with a direct antispasmodic action on smooth muscle. It is included at a low dose (2.5 mg per 5 ml) with antacids and simeticone in Kolanticon Gel (Peckforton). Dicycloverine tablets and syrup (Merbentyl [Florizel]) are not marketed for over-the-counter sale but may be supplied without prescription, provided the maximum single dose is 10 mg and the maximum daily dose is 60 mg.

Contraindications and interactions

All products containing antimuscarinics are contraindicated in patients with glaucoma; those containing tertiary amines should also be avoided by patients with prostatic hypertrophy, myasthenia gravis or thyrotoxicosis. It is generally advisable to avoid the use of products containing antimuscarinics in elderly patients. Indigestion preparations containing antimuscarinic antispasmodics, especially tertiary amines, should not be recommended to patients taking medicines that exert antimuscarinic side-effects; these include tricyclic antidepressants, monoamine oxidase inhibitors, antihistamines and phenothiazine antipsychotics. The effects of sublingual tablets may also be reduced because of the reduction in salivary secretion caused by antimuscarinics. Antimuscarinics will also antagonise the effect of motility stimulants such as metoclopramide and domperidone, which are sometimes used to treat dyspepsia.

Products

- Atropine
  - Actonorm powder
    Wallace

- Dicycloverine
  - Kolanticon gel
    Peckforton

Actonorm and Kolanticon Gel are compound preparations containing antacids as well as an antispasmodic.

TREATMENT – H₂-ANTAGONISTS

Compounds available

Compounds available are:

- famotidine
- ranitidine.

Mode of action

Histamine is thought to be the most important mediator of gastric acid secretion through activation of receptors on parietal cells. It stimulates the production of a protein kinase, which in turn activates parietal cell proton pumps, the enzyme hydrogen/potassium adenosine triphosphatase (H^+/K^+ ATPase), to secrete hydrogen ions into the stomach. H_2-receptor antagonists interfere with this mechanism by occupying receptor sites on the parietal cells, blocking the action of histamine. H_1-antagonists, used in the treatment of hay fever and allergic reactions, are of little use in controlling gastric acid secretion.

H_2-antagonists have been used extensively for the treatment of peptic ulcer and related conditions for about 30 years, and the evidence of research and trials running into hundreds of published papers confirms their effectiveness and safety as prescription medicines. Much less information is available about H_2-antagonists as non-prescription products. Such trials as have been published indicate that H_2-antagonists are more effective treatments than antacids for non-ulcer dyspepsia.[7]

H_2-antagonists exert their effect for longer than antacids, as their action is not limited by the length of contact with the stomach contents. Ranitidine reaches peak plasma levels about 1 hour after ingestion and the elimination half-life is 2–3 hours. Peak plasma levels of famotidine are reached in about 2 hours and the half-life is up to 4 hours. With both drugs, acid secretion is inhibited for much longer; famotidine provides relief for up to 9 hours after a dose, reflected in the twice-daily dosage.

H_2-antagonists suffer the disadvantage in relation to antacids that they do not act quickly. For both rapid and extended relief, therefore, an antacid and an H_2-antagonist can be taken together; the action of H_2-antagonists is not inhibited in the presence of antacids. A combination product containing calcium carbonate, magnesium hydroxide and famotidine (Pepcidtwo [McNeil]) is available.

There is no indication that either H_2-antagonist is more effective than the other at relieving symptoms of dyspepsia.

Uses

H_2-antagonists are licensed for the symptomatic relief of heartburn, indigestion and acid indigestion, and also for prevention of indigestion and heartburn associated with food and drink consumption. They can therefore be taken in advance of consuming food or drink that is known to provoke dyspepsia.

H_2-antagonists are licensed for use for a maximum of 2 weeks. Although this requirement has been introduced for products licensed relatively recently, it reflects a principle that should be applied to all medicines sold for the treatment of indigestion. Patients should be referred to a doctor for further investigation if indigestion symptoms persist after 2 weeks' treatment with any over-the-counter medicine.

Dosage

- **Famotidine:** 10 mg for symptomatic relief or 1 hour before consuming food or drink that causes symptoms; maximum dose 20 mg in 24 hours.
- **Ranitidine:** 75 mg for symptomatic relief, followed by 75 mg 1 hour later if symptoms persist; maximum dose 300 mg in 24 hours.
- All products are restricted to use in adults and children over 16 years of age.
- **Nizatidine** has been classified as a Pharmacy medicine at a dose of 75 mg for adults and children over 16 years of age. The maximum dose is 150 mg daily for a maximum of 14 days. Currently there is no 75 mg dosage form available.

Cautions and interactions

H$_2$-antagonists are well tolerated and the incidence of side-effects is low. They should not be sold to patients taking non-steroidal anti-inflammatory drugs, as these may mask the symptoms of developing peptic ulcer. H$_2$-antagonists are not licensed for sale to pregnant or breastfeeding women.

The activity of drugs that require an acid medium for absorption may be reduced by H$_2$-antagonists; both ketoconazole and itraconazole are known to be so affected.

Products

Products are licensed as Pharmacy medicines (P) or General sale list (GSL), as indicated below.

- Famotidine
    — Pepcidtwo chewable tablets (also contains calcium carbonate and magnesium hydroxide) (GSL)
    McNeil

- Ranitidine
    — Gavilast (6 and 12 tablets packs; GSL)
    — Gavilast P (24 and 48 tablets packs; P)
    Reckitt Benckiser
    — Ranzac tablets (GSL)
    LPC
    — Zantac 75 Relief tablets (6 and 12 tablets packs; GSL)
    — Zantac 75 tablets (24 tablet pack; P)
    GSK Consumer Healthcare

TREATMENT – OMEPRAZOLE

Mode of action

Omeprazole is a selective proton pump inhibitor; it directly inhibits the H^+/K^+ ATPase of the parietal cells of the stomach responsible for gastric acid secretion, and blocks the terminal secretion process of gastric acid. Omeprazole has a more prolonged effect on acid suppression than H_2-antagonists and a short course can give several weeks' remission from recurrent attacks.[8]

Uses

Heartburn is a chronic, intermittent, relapsing disorder of varying frequency and severity. Although there is usually no underlying pathology, sufferers can experience recurrent attacks, including at night, which can be distressing and negatively affect quality of life. Omeprazole is primarily indicated for these patients.

Dosage

The initial dose is two 10 mg tablets once daily, swallowed whole before a meal with plenty of liquid, until symptoms subside. Thereafter, a dose of 10 mg once daily can be taken, increasing to 20 mg if symptoms return. If no relief is obtained within 2 weeks or if continuous treatment for more than 4 weeks is required to relieve symptoms, the patient should be referred to their doctor. Patients should be advised that omeprazole does not provide instant relief from symptoms, although improvement is usually felt within 24 hours. An antacid preparation can be taken initially together with omeprazole to provide quick relief, but H_2 antagonists should not be taken concomitantly.

Cautions and interactions

Omeprazole is licensed for non-prescription use in adults aged 18 years and over. It should not be used by pregnant or breastfeeding women.

The medicine should not be supplied, and the patient should be referred to their doctor, if any of the following apply:

- an indigestion or heartburn remedy has had to be taken continuously for 4 or more weeks in order to control symptoms
- age over 45 years with new or recently changed symptoms
- any symptom that might indicate a more serious gastrointestinal condition
- any previous gastric ulcer or surgery, jaundice or any other significant medical condition (including hepatic and renal impairment).

Omeprazole is metabolised in the liver by the cytochrome P450 isoenzymes, and significant interactions are possible with anticoagulants and antiepileptics. Concomitant use with cilostazol should also be avoided, as omeprazole increases its plasma concentration. Absorption of ketoconazole and itraconazole may be delayed because of reduced stomach acidity. The manufacturer also recommends caution with diazepam and digoxin.

Product

- Zanprol tablets
  GSK Consumer Healthcare

TREATMENT – DOMPERIDONE

Mode of action

Domperidone is a dopamine D_2-receptor antagonist; its mechanism of action and prokinetic and antiemetic properties are similar to those of metoclopramide. Unlike metoclopramide, domperidone does not cross the blood–brain barrier readily and acts primarily on dopamine receptors in the gastrointestinal tract. It has a high affinity for the tissues of the oesophagus, stomach and small intestine, where it acts to enhance gastric and oesophageal sphincter tone, gastric emptying and propulsion of intestinal contents.

Uses

Domperidone is licensed for the treatment of dysmotility symptoms of dyspepsia, including sensations of fullness, bloating, 'heavy stomach', trapped wind, belching and nausea. A number of clinical studies generally indicate that prokinetic drugs are effective for the above symptoms.[7]

Dosage

The recommended dose is one 10 mg tablet three times daily and at night, when required. The drug is licensed for use in adults of 16 years and over.

Cautions and interactions

Domperidone is not recommended during pregnancy or breastfeeding. It should also be avoided by patients with any underlying gastric pathology, those with impaired hepatic or renal function or with prolactinoma. Risk of raised serum prolactin and central side-effects, such as extrapyramidal effects, are extremely low at over-the-counter dosages but pharmacists should advise patients against prolonged use.

There is theoretical potential for interaction between domperidone and several types of drug, although no problems appear to have occurred in practice. Opioid analgesics and antimuscarinic drugs may antagonise the effect of domperidone; paracetamol absorption may be enhanced; the hypoprolactinaemic effects of bromocriptine and cabergoline may be antagonised.

Product

- Motilium 10 tablets
  McNeil

PRODUCT SELECTION POINTS

- Despite the availability of histamine H_2-antagonists and omemprazole as Pharmacy medicines, antacids generally remain the first choice of treatment for indigestion. Evidence from trials and widespread use has shown antacids to be effective. They have the advantage of cheapness and rapid action, although their action is less prolonged than that of H_2-antagonists or omeprazole.
- Antacid preparations containing both aluminium and magnesium salts are a good choice as they are effective and long acting, and are not absorbed to a significant extent. This combination also minimises potential adverse effects from either component and balances the constipating action of aluminium against the laxative effect of magnesium salts.
- Regular use of antacids containing significant amounts of sodium should be avoided by patients with hypertension and other cardiovascular problems, and by pregnant women.
- Many antacid preparations have a high sugar content, which should be considered when recommending products to patients with diabetes.
- Antacid preparations containing bismuth salicylate should not be recommended to patients who are sensitive to aspirin.

- Antacids are more effective if taken about 1 hour after eating. Because of interactions in the stomach between antacids and many other drugs, a 2-hour gap should be left between a dose of an antacid and another medicine.
- Liquid antacid preparations are faster acting and may be more effective than tablets, but tablets are more convenient.
- Preparations containing alginates are worth trying for symptoms associated with reflux oesophagitis if plain antacids are ineffective. H_2-antagonists may be more effective, particularly for night-time symptoms.
- Products containing antiflatulents can be tried if bloating or distension complicate indigestion, although there is no conclusive evidence that these combinations are more effective than antacids alone.
- Products containing antispasmodics may be worth trying to treat symptoms of colic or cramp associated with indigestion. However, they should not be recommended to elderly patients, and the wide range of drugs that they interact with should be taken into account.
- H_2-antagonists are effective for treating indigestion, including heartburn, but are more expensive than antacids. They may be best reserved for patients whose symptoms are not adequately relieved by antacids.
- Omeprazole appears to be an effective treatment for recurrent heartburn.
- Domperidone can be used for dysmotility symptoms.
- A patient who still has indigestion after 2 weeks' treatment with any indigestion medicine should be referred to a doctor.

PRODUCT RECOMMENDATIONS

- For indigestion uncomplicated by additional symptoms – a combination antacid containing magnesium and aluminium salts.
- To carry around for occasional use – tablets as above, or containing calcium carbonate.
- For heartburn, reflux oesophagitis unresponsive to simple antacids (but not for pregnant women or elderly or hypertensive patients) – an H_2-antagonist or an alginate-containing antacid preparation.
- For pregnant women (usually last trimester), and elderly and hypertensive patients with heartburn – a sodium-free or low-sodium antacid preparation containing an alginate.
- For indigestion not adequately relieved by antacids – an H_2-antagonist, with careful monitoring of the situation.
- For recurrent heartburn – omeprazole, with monitoring of the situation.

The above recommendations are made on the assumption that the possibility of a potentially serious gastrointestinal condition has been eliminated.

REFERENCES

1. Ching CK, Lam SK. Antacids. Indications and limitations. *Drugs* 1994; 47: 305–317.
2. Mandel KG, Daggy BP, Brodie DA, Jacoby HI. Review article: alginate-raft formulations in the treatment of heartburn and acid reflux. *Aliment Pharmacol Ther* 2000; 14: 669–690.
3. Goves J, Oldring JK, Kerr D, *e al*. First line treatment with omeprazole provides an effective and superior alternative strategy in the management of dyspepsia compared to antacid/alginate liquid: a multicentre study in general practice. *Aliment Pharmacol Ther* 1998; 12: 147–157.
4. Krska J, John DN, Hansford D, Kennedy EJ. Drug utilization evaluation of nonprescription H2–receptor antagonists and alginate-containing preparations for dyspepsia. *Br J Clin Pharmacol* 2000; 49: 363–368.
5. Dimethicone for gastrointestinal symptoms? *Drug Ther Bull* 1986; 24: 21–22.

6. Simethicone for gastrointestinal gas. *Med Lett Drugs Ther* 1996; 38: 57–58.

7. Moayyedi P, Soo S, Deeks J, *et al.* Pharmacological interventions for non-ulcer dyspepsia. *The Cochrane Library,* issue 1. Chichester, UK: John Wiley & Sons, 2005 (www.thecochranelibrary.com).

8. Bardhan KD, Muller-Lissner S, Bigard MA, *et al.* Symptomatic gastro-oesophageal reflux disease: double blind controlled study of intermittent treatment with omeprazole or ranitidine. The European Study Group. *BMJ* 1999; 20: 502–507.

Insect bites and stings

Insect bites and stings differ in the chemical composition of their constituents and in the type of reaction they provoke. Insect bites often go unnoticed at the time, and their effects may not be felt for some time afterwards but can then last for several days. Stings are felt immediately and the pain and discomfort they cause often subsides within minutes or hours.

Bites

Insects usually bite in order to gain access to the victim's blood supply to feed on it. The skin is punctured and the insect's saliva is secreted into the dermis. The saliva contains enzymes or other agents to liquefy the blood in order to facilitate its flow back through the insect's feeding apparatus. It may also contain a local anaesthetic, so that the bite goes undetected by the victim and allows the insect to feed undisturbed. The reaction produced by the bite is essentially an irritant dermatitis provoked by the insect's saliva.

Stings

Insect stings are primarily weapons, either of attack when used to incapacitate prey, or of defence when a threat is perceived, and their effect is intended to be immediate. The pain and inflammation of a bee or wasp sting is caused by the direct pharmacological effects of its constituents. These include: histamine and other biogenic amines; toxic polypeptides, including melittin, which has a haemolytic effect; apamin, which is neurotoxic; mast cell degranulating peptide, which causes further release of histamine; plus enzymes such as hyaluronidase and phospholipase, which break down intercellular tissue cement and assist penetration of the venom into the tissues.

Preparations marketed for the treatment of bites and stings contain:

- antihistamines
- local anaesthetics
- astringents
- soothing constituents.

Preparations are generally intended to suppress cutaneous sensory receptors. Hydrocortisone is also licensed for the treatment of insect bites.

Antihistamines

As one of the principal components of insect stings is histamine, and as histamine is also one of the principal mediators of the inflammatory response to bites, treatment with antihistamines, which competitively block histamine H_1-receptors, seems logical. Several topical products containing antihistamines are licensed for treatment of the pain, itching and inflammation associated with bites and stings. However, topical antihistamines have been criticised as not being very effective.[1] They are also liable to cause sensitisation, and for this reason their use is restricted to a maximum of two or three applications per day for no longer than 3 days.

Oral antihistamines are more likely than topical preparations to bring sustained and effective relief. Non-sedating compounds are preferable, being as effective as the older antihistamines for peripherally mediated reactions but are not associated with central sedating and antimuscarinic side-effects. (For further information on antihistamines, see the chapter on Hay fever.)

Some patients develop an allergic sensitivity to bites and suffer quite severe local reactions. Such patients should be advised to keep a supply of antihistamines with them, ready to take in case they are bitten, as well as taking precautions against being bitten. A few individuals develop severe anaphylaxis to stings; they may be prescribed adrenaline (epinephrine) 1:1000 injection to keep at hand for intramuscular or subcutaneous use if they are stung.

Products

- Diphenhydramine
  - Benadryl Skin Allergy Relief cream and lotion
    Pfizer Consumer Healthcare
  - Histergan cream
    Norma Chemicals

- Mepyramine
  - Anthisan Bite and Sting cream
  - Anthisan Plus Sting Relief spray (also contains benzocaine)
    both *Sanofi-Aventis*
  - Wasp-Eze spray (also contains benzocaine)
    SSL International

All of the products listed above are also licensed for the treatment of allergic skin reactions.

Crotamiton

Crotamiton is not an antihistamine but has antipruritic properties and can be used for bites and stings; it is claimed to have a prolonged action of 6–10 hours following application. (Crotamiton is also licensed for the treatment of allergic skin reactions.)

Products

- Eurax cream and lotion
- Eurax HC cream (also contains hydrocortisone)
  both *Novartis Consumer Health*

Local anaesthetics

The effectiveness of local anaesthetics in the treatment of bites and stings is debatable. A US Food and Drug Administration advisory panel concluded that products containing them are safe and effective, but claims have also been made that the concentrations found in non-prescription products are insufficient to produce adequate pain relief.[2] Sensitisation on prolonged usage is an acknowledged problem and licensing restrictions on the length of use take account of this.

Spray formulations may be more effective than creams or lotions as they contain higher concentrations of local anaesthetic. They are likely to be most useful immediately after a bite or sting because they will produce relief, although short-lived, when the pain is most intense. The cooling effect produced by the evaporation of the propellant will also contribute to the pain relief. (For further information on local anaesthetics, see chapter on Haemorrhoids.)

Products

- Benzocaine
    - Anthisan Plus Sting Relief spray (also contains mepyramine)
      Sanofi-Aventis
    - Lanacane cream
      Coombe International
    - Solarcaine cream, lotion and spray
      Schering-Plough
    - Wasp-Eze spray (also contains mepyramine)
      SSL International

- Lidocaine
    - Dermidex dermatological cream
      Thornton & Ross

- Tetracaine
  — Anethaine cream
    Torbet

Hydrocortisone

The usefulness of hydrocortisone cream for bites may be limited by being restricted to two applications daily, as more frequent application may be necessary to sustain relief. It is not licensed for use in children under 10 years of age.

Products

For products, see chapter on Irritant and allergic dermatitis.

Calamine/zinc oxide

Calamine is naturally occurring basic zinc carbonate with ferric oxide, which imparts the characteristic pink colour. It is mildly astringent and its soothing antipruritic action is due to the large surface area and porous nature of its particles, which promote the evaporation of water from the preparations in which it is formulated, with a consequent cooling effect. Calamine Lotion BP also contains 0.5% phenol as a preservative, which has an incidental local anaesthetic action and contributes to its effectiveness. It is a popular preparation for treating urticaria and pruritus from many causes, including insect bites. It is cheap and there are few restrictions on its use. Zinc oxide has similar properties to calamine.

Products

- Calamine
  — Calamine Cream, Aqueous BP

case in doubt. Calamine lotion may be the best topical treatment for bites, as it is an effective antipruritic, can be applied as frequently as required and is cheap.

- For bites, oral antihistamines are likely to provide more effective and prolonged relief than either topical hydrocortisone or topical antihistamines, although their action is not immediate. Non-sedating compounds should be as effective as the older, sedating ones and are not associated with the latters' side-effects. The best overall approach may be use of a topical preparation immediately plus an oral antihistamine to maintain relief.
- A spray presentation containing a local anaesthetic may be the best initial treatment for stings, but early application is essential for optimum response. Continued relief can be provided as for bites.

DUCT RECOMMENDATIONS

- For insect bites – hydrocortisone cream or ointment or calamine lotion, and an oral antihistamine if necessary.
- For stings – a spray containing a local anaesthetic used promptly, and an oral antihistamine if necessary.

RENCES

1.   Palop V, Pastor C, Rubio E, Martinez-Mir I. [Topical antihistaminics. Is their use justified?] [Article in Spanish] *Aten Primaria* 1996; 18: 47–48.
2.   Wilson H. Dermatitis from anaesthetic ointments. *Practitioner* 1966; 197: 673–677.
3.   Frohman IG. Treatment of physalia stings. *JAMA* 1966; 197: 733.

- — Calamine Lotion BP
- — Lactocalamine creme and lotion
  Schering-Plough

- Zinc oxide
  - — Benadryl Skin Allergy Relief cream an
    Pfizer Consumer Healthcare
  - — Lactocalamine cream and lotion
    Schering-Plough

Ammonia solution

Ammonia has been claimed to have a neutralising
stings. It is frequently recommended in consume
websites and there is a documented report of the su
matic Ammonia Spirit to treat bathers who had
tuguese men-of-war jelly fish; otherwise, however,
no objective evidence of its effectiveness.[3]

Product

There is only one product:

- After Bite applicator pen
  Ardern

PRODUCT SELECTION POINTS

- Although hydrocortisone cream and ointme
  the treatment of insect bite reactions, their e
  limited by restrictions on the frequency of ap
  applies to topical antihistamines, the efficacy

PI

R

Irritable bowel syndrome

Irritable bowel syndrome (IBS) is a chronic motility disorder of the colon.

There is no demonstrable organic cause for IBS. It is characterised by a range of symptoms which may include abdominal pain (either colicky or dull and aching), diarrhoea or constipation (or both alternately), abdominal distension and flatulence, together with non-intestinal symptoms such as headache and fatigue. Symptoms are often exacerbated by stress, anxiety or depression. As the cause cannot be determined, treatment is symptomatic. Much of the reported efficacy of treatments has been ascribed to placebo effect.[1]

A number of preparations are believed to have a direct relaxant effect on intestinal smooth muscle, are available without prescription and are licensed specifically for the treatment of IBS. Ispaghula husk is also used (it is also licensed for other indications). The preparations are:

- alverine citrate
- hyoscine butylbromide
- mebeverine hydrochloride
- peppermint oil
- ispaghula husk.

Alverine citrate

Alverine is a non-antimuscarinic selective antispasmodic that acts directly on smooth muscle; it is used for the treatment of pain and smooth muscle spasm in IBS. There were few side-effects reported during the 30 years it was available as a prescription medicine and it was reclassified as a Pharmacy medicine in 1998. It has no known interactions. A randomised controlled trial[2] found it to be no better than placebo at relieving the symptoms of IBS.

The recommended dose for adults and children over 12 years is one or two 60 mg capsules up to three times daily. It is not con-traindicated during pregnancy and breastfeeding, but caution is advised in the first trimester of pregnancy. The manufacturer recom-mends that the drug should be supplied only to patients who have had IBS diagnosed by a doctor.

Product

- Spasmonal capsules
  Norgine

Hyoscine butylbromide

Hyoscine butylbromide is an antimuscarinic antispasmodic. It is a hydrophilic quaternary ammonium compound that is poorly absorbed from the gut and is claimed to act directly on it; any drug that is absorbed does not readily cross the blood–brain barrier. Never-theless, antimuscarinic side-effects have been very occasionally reported and hyoscine butylbromide is contraindicated in patients with glaucoma. Caution is also advised for men with prostate prob-lems, the elderly and pregnant women. A double-blind, randomised, parallel-group trial carried out by the manufacturer of Buscopan found that it was suitable for the treatment of IBS.[3] The recommended dosage is three to eight 10 mg tablets daily, in divided doses, for adults, and 30 mg daily for children aged 6–12 years.

Product

- Buscopan IBS Relief tablets
  Boehringer Ingelheim

Mebeverine hydrochloride

Mebeverine is a musculotropic antispasmodic which is claimed to act directly on the smooth muscle of the intestine without affecting normal gut motility. Like alverine, it has no antimuscarinic side-effects and no contraindications or interactions with other drugs. A clinical trial[4] found mebeverine to be no better than placebo and inferior to wheat bran in the treatment of IBS.

Mebeverine hydrochloride is licensed for use in adults and children over 10 years of age; it should be used in pregnancy only under medical supervision. The dosage is 135 mg up to three times daily, taken 20 minutes before meals.

Product

- Colofac IBS tablets
  Solvay

Peppermint oil

Menthol, the principal constituent of peppermint oil, has been shown to have a relaxant action on smooth muscle similar to that of calcium channel antagonists. The oil acts directly on the colon; evidence as to its effectiveness in treating IBS is conflicting, however.[5,6]

Peppermint oil is available as enteric-coated capsules containing 0.2 mL oil. The recommended dosage for adults is one or two capsules three times a day, preferably before food; it may be taken after food, but not immediately after. The capsules should not be chewed, as peppermint oil can cause irritation of the mouth and oesophagus; in addition, the drug would be dispersed before reaching the colon. Heartburn sufferers may, in any case, experience an exacerbation of symptoms even when the capsules are taken correctly. Peppermint-oil capsules are not contraindicated in pregnancy or breastfeeding, although the usual precautions should be observed.

Products

- Colpermin capsules
  Pfizer Consumer Health

- Mintec capsules
  Shire

Ispaghula husk

Ispaghula husk is licensed for the treatment of IBS as well as for constipation and diarrhoea. The balance of opinion appears to be slightly in favour of ispaghula husk being effective in the treatment of IBS. One systematic review[7] found there was no evidence that fibre was effective in the relief of abdominal pain in IBS, and that insoluble fibre (which includes ispaghula) in some cases worsened the clinical outcome. One reviewer[8] has stated that ispaghula can increase stool frequency and help pain but that it may aggravate bloating. Two double-blind, placebo-controlled trials[9,10] found that that it significantly improved overall well-being in patients with IBS. Dosage is as for constipation. (See chapter on Constipation.)

PRODUCT SELECTION POINTS

- All of the drugs discussed above have a long history of use for IBS, but convincing evidence of their efficacy from clinical trials is lacking. No treatment can therefore be recommended above any other.
- As psychological factors are likely to contribute to IBS in many cases, a placebo effect could play a large part in the perceived effectiveness of any treatment.

PRODUCT RECOMMENDATIONS

A successful treatment for an individual patient may be found by trial and error. Before making any recommendation, the pharmacist should ensure that the patient has been diagnosed by a doctor as suffering from IBS.

REFERENCES

1.   Fennerty MB. Traditional therapies for irritable bowel syndrome: an evidence-based appraisal. *Rev Gastroenterol Disord* 2003; 3 (Suppl 2): S18–S24.
2.   Mitchell SA, Mee AS, Smith GD, *et al.* Alverine citrate fails to relieve the symptoms of irritable bowel syndrome: results of a double-blind, randomized, placebo-controlled trial. *Aliment Pharmacol Ther* 2002; 16: 1187–1195.
3.   Schafer E, Ewe K. [The treatment of irritable colon. Efficacy and tolerance of buscopan plus, buscopan, paracetamol and placebo in ambulatory patients with irritable colon] [Article in German] *Fortschr Med* 1990; 108: 488–492.
4.   Kruis W, Weinzierl M, Schussler P, Holl J. Comparison of the therapeutic effect of wheat bran, mebeverine and placebo in patients with the irritable bowel syndrome. *Digestion* 1986; 34: 196–201.
5.   Pittler MH, Ernst E. Peppermint oil for irritable bowel syndrome: a critical review and metaanalysis. *Am J Gastroenterol* 1998; 93: 1131–1135.
6.   Liu JH, Chen GH, Yeh HZ, *et al.* Enteric-coated peppermint-oil capsules in the treatment of irritable bowel syndrome: a prospective, randomized trial. *J Gastroenterol* 1997; 32: 765–768.
7.   Bijkerk CJ, Muris JW, Knottnerus JA, *et al.* Systematic review: the role of different types of fibre in the treatment of irritable bowel syndrome. *Aliment Pharmacol Ther* 2004; 19: 245–251.
8.   Spiller RC. Treatment of irritable bowel syndrome. *Curr Treat Options Gastroenterol* 2003 ; 6: 329–337.
9.   Prior A, Whorwell PJ. Double blind study of ispaghula in irritable bowel syndrome. *Gut* 1987; 28: 1510–1513.
10. Jalihal A, Kurian G. Ispaghula therapy in irritable bowel syndrome: improvement in overall well-being is related to reduction in bowel dissatisfaction. *J Gastroenterol Hepatol* 1990; 5: 507–513.

Irritant and allergic dermatitis and mild eczema

Dermatitis and eczema are terms used interchangeably by dermatologists to describe a range of inflammatory skin conditions, the principal symptoms of which are dryness, erythema and itch, often with weeping and crusting. However, it has become conventional to apply the term eczema to conditions with an endogenous cause in atopic individuals and dermatitis to reactions to external agents.

CAUSES

Atopic eczema

Atopic eczema is a chronic fluctuating inflammatory condition of the skin with no known cause, although there is often a genetic link and a family history of allergic sensitivity. It affects 5–15% of schoolchildren and 2–10% of adults. It usually resolves spontaneously by 30 years of age, although the skin may remain sensitive to irritant agents. The rash of atopic eczema usually starts on the face and then spreads to the hands and flexural sites around the body; the exact pattern of distribution depends on age.

Irritant dermatitis

Irritant dermatitis results from contact with substances that cause direct chemical damage to the skin, and can occur on the first exposure to a strong irritant or on repeated exposure to a milder one. It is commonly associated with occupational use. Examples of irritant agents include: detergents and household cleaning materials; hair tinting and perming products; acids, alkalis, industrial solvents, oils and plastics used by textile workers, car mechanics, woodworkers, decorators and builders; and fertilisers and soil, which florists and agricultural workers come into contact with. The reaction is confined to the area of contact with the causative agent.

Allergic contact dermatitis

Allergic contact dermatitis results from hypersensitivity to a sensitising agent, which can occur after just a couple of exposures or may take many years of repeated exposure to develop. The rash may appear at, or away from, the site of contact. Once established, sensitivity generally remains for life. Sensitising agents include: rubber in household gloves and footwear; nickel in costume jewellery, zips, bra clips, belt buckles and coins; resins used in glues; ingredients of cosmetics and topical medications; plants, particularly primula and chrysanthemum; and chromates in paints and cement.

TREATMENT

Hydrocortisone cream and ointment

The principal problems in atopic eczema are skin dryness and itch over widespread areas, and the mainstays of treatment are hydrating agents and soothing emollients. Topical corticosteroids are used to treat severe flare-ups, and systemic sedative antihistamines may be given to alleviate itching, particularly at night. Atopic eczema should be treated under medical supervision, although hydrocortisone cream is licensed for the treatment of mild-to-moderate eczema (see below), and most antihistamines are available without prescription.

Community pharmacists are likely to be asked for advice and to provide treatment for irritation caused by contact dermatitis, the standard treatment for which is hydrocortisone cream or ointment. (For treatment of Eczema, see also chapter on Dry skin conditions.)

Mode of action

The mechanism of the local anti-inflammatory action of corticosteroids is described in the chapter on Mouth ulcers.

In creams and ointments for non-prescription use, only hydrocortisone as the free alcohol and hydrocortisone-21-acetate are permitted. These compounds have only mild potency, a short duration of activity, weak side-effects and a better safety profile compared with other topical corticosteroids. Also, unlike more potent corticosteroids, hydrocortisone does not affect protein synthesis in human skin and is therefore unlikely to cause antiproliferative side-effects such as thinning of the skin and telangiectasis (dilatation of superficial blood capillaries).

Indications

In 1987, hydrocortisone cream and ointment, up to a concentration of 1%, were licensed for sale without prescription from pharmacies for the treatment of inflammation and pruritus associated with irritant and allergic contact dermatitis and insect-bite reactions, but not for atopic eczema, for which hydrocortisone remained a Prescription-only medicine. These restricted indications caused difficulties, as patients did not understand why they could buy hydrocortisone for contact dermatitis but not for eczema, even when their doctor had recommended purchase.

When hydrocortisone was first reclassified as a Pharmacy medicine, there was considerable opposition from some medical quarters, concern being expressed over safety once it was freed from prescription control. One of the major fears was that misuse might lead to systemic absorption sufficient to cause adrenal suppression. However, experience has proved hydrocortisone to be safe as a non-prescription medicine, and in 1995 the licensed indications were extended to include mild-to-moderate eczema.

Hydrocortisone has also since been licensed in combination products with the antipruritic crotamiton and with the antifungals, clotrimazole and miconazole; indications for the hydrocortisone-plus-antifungal combinations were further extended to athlete's foot and candidal intertrigo. Haemorrhoidal preparations containing hydrocortisone are also now licensed as Pharmacy medicines.

Use, cautions and restrictions

Hydrocortisone cream and ointment should be applied sparingly once or twice daily for a maximum of 7 days. The licensing conditions restrict application to a 'small area', presumably in order to limit the potential for widespread application in atopic eczema and any possible risk of skin damage or systemic absorption.

Preparations should not be used on the eyes or face, although they may be applied to the ear lobes, which are often the site of allergic contact dermatitis caused by nickel in costume jewellery earrings. Use on anogenital areas is not permitted, although haemorrhoidal preparations containing hydrocortisone are licensed for rectal use.

Hydrocortisone cream or ointment should not be applied to any infections of the skin, including athlete's foot (although clotrimazole-with-hydrocortisone cream and miconazole-with-hydrocortisone cream are licensed for this indication), acne or cold sores, as symptoms may be masked while the infection is allowed to progress and natural immune reactions may be suppressed by the steroid. Preparations should not be applied to ulcerated, broken or weeping skin, or used with occlusive dressings, because of the risk of absorption.

In addition to the restrictions relating to application, hydrocortisone cream and ointment is not licensed for use in children under 10 years of age, or during pregnancy or breastfeeding.

Products

The following products contain 1% hydrocortisone or hydrocortisone acetate and are licensed for sale without prescription:

- Hc45 cream
  Crookes

- Lanacort cream and ointment
  Coombe International

- Zenoxone cream
  Biorex

- Dermacort cream (0.1% hydrocortisone in a formulation designed to provide equivalent activity to 1% Hydrocortisone Cream BP)
  Sankyo

- Eurax HC cream (0.25% hydrocortisone with 10% crotamiton)
  Novartis Consumer Health

Note that packs of hydrocortisone cream and ointment (1%) licensed as prescription-only medicines may not be sold without prescription as they do not comply with the labelling requirements for over-the-counter sale.

Clobetasone butyrate cream

Clobetasone butyrate 0.05% cream was reclassified as a Pharmacy medicine in 2001. Clobetasone butyrate is a moderately potent corticosteroid, and is licensed for the short-term treatment and control of patches of eczema and dermatitis, including atopic eczema and primary irritant and allergic dermatitis. It is more effective than hydrocortisone for flare-ups of eczema, and will generally break the 'itch–scratch cycle' before it takes hold. The licensing conditions and restrictions are generally as for hydrocortisone cream, but the product may be used for children under 12 years of age on the advice of a doctor.

Clobetasone butyrate cream should not be used on the same area of skin for more than two 1-week treatment periods within 3 months, or for the treatment of psoriasis or seborrhoeic eczema.

Product

- Eumovate Eczema and Dermatitis cream
  GSK Consumer Healthcare

Efficacy of hydrocortisone and clobetasone

A systematic review[1] of 83 trials of topical corticosteroids for atopic eczema concluded that they were effective and produced few adverse effects, but that there is a large treatment effect and the type of vehicle used may enhance efficacy. There appear to be no comparative trials of hydrocortisone versus clobetasone, although both appear to be more effective than other treatments.[2,3] Some doubt regarding the efficacy of topical corticosteroids in irritant contact dermatitis has been expressed.[4]

PRODUCT SELECTION POINTS

- Hydrocortisone cream and ointment are licensed for sale without prescription for irritant and allergic dermatitis. They are safe and effective when used in accordance with the licensing restrictions.
- Hydrocortisone cream is also licensed for sale without prescription for mild-to-moderate eczema. However, licensing restrictions limit application to small areas only and prevent use on the face and in children under 10 years of age, precluding most of its uses in atopic eczema. The condition should be treated wherever possible with emollients (see chapter on Dry skin).
- Clobetasone butyrate 0.05% cream is available for flare-ups of atopic eczema.

PRODUCT RECOMMENDATIONS

- For contact and allergic dermatitis – hydrocortisone cream or ointment.
- For flare-ups of atopic eczema – clobetasone butyrate 0.05% cream.

REFERENCES

1. Hoare C, Li Wan Po A, Williams H. Systematic review of treatments for atopic eczema. *Health Technol Assess* 2000; 4(37).
2. Morley N, Fry L, Walker S. Clinical evaluation of clobetasone butyrate in the treatment of children with atopic eczema, and its effect on plasma corticosteroid levels. *Curr Med Res Opin* 1976; 4: 223–228.
3. Korting HC, Schafer-Korting M, Klovekorn W, *et al*. Comparative efficacy of hamamelis distillate and hydrocortisone cream in atopic eczema. *Eur J Clin Pharmacol* 1995; 48: 461–465.
4. Levin C, Zhai H, Bashir S, *et al*. Efficacy of corticosteroids in acute experimental irritant contact dermatitis? *Skin Res Technol* 2001; 7: 214–218.

Migraine

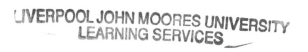

Migraine is a periodically occurring syndrome of which headache is a principal component. The frequency of attacks varies between individuals, from several per week to just a few in the course of a lifetime. Overall prevalence of the condition is about 10%, with three times as many women as men affected. Attacks may be preceded by a prodromal stage in which there are vague changes in mood and appetite, and in about a quarter of sufferers by an aura in which clear neurological symptoms such as visual, motor or sensory disturbances are experienced for up to an hour before the headache begins. Migraine in which there is an aura is described as 'classical' migraine; migraine without aura is known as 'common' migraine. The headache is often pulsatile and initially unilateral, although it may later spread across the head. It is often associated with nausea and vomiting and, in classical migraine, with photophobia and phonophobia. Attacks last 4–72 hours, and can be disabling.

CAUSES

The causes of migraine are still not known with certainty, but symptoms of aura may be caused by vasoconstriction in the brain and the subsequent headache may be the result of vasodilatation. Aura symptoms have also been ascribed to neuronal dysfunction. It is also thought that a hypothalamic trigger may cause periodic overactivity of the trigeminal pain pathways.

TREATMENT

Until recently, the only non-prescription treatments available were the analgesics aspirin, ibuprofen and paracetamol, co-formulated in one product with codeine and an antihistamine to counteract nausea and vomiting. In 1999, a co-formulation of paracetamol with a vasoconstrictor was reclassified from Prescription-only medicine to Pharmacy medicine, and in 2001 prochlorperazine was licensed for over-the-counter sale for treatment of nausea and vomiting associated with migraine. A consultation on the reclassification of sumatriptan and zolmitriptan was issued by the Medicines and Health Care Regulatory Authority in August 2005. Sumatriptan was reclassified in May 2006, but the reclassification of zolmitriptan is still awaited. Progress will be reported via the 6-monthly updates on the Pharmaceutical Press website (see Preface).

Buclizine

Buclizine 6.25 mg is included in Migraleve (Pfizer Consumer Health-care), for its anti-emetic action. Migraleve is licensed specifically for the treatment of migraine. Migraleve Pink tablets contain buclizine together with paracetamol 500 mg and codeine 8 mg. For adults, two tablets are taken as an initial dose as soon as an attack starts or is felt to be imminent, followed by two Migraleve Yellow tablets, which contain only paracetamol and codeine, 4 hourly thereafter if necessary. The dose for children aged 10–14 years is one tablet. The product is not licensed for use in children under 10 years of age and is not recommended in pregnancy, but can be taken by breastfeeding women.

In a small double-blind, randomised, cross-over trial,[1] Migraleve was found to be significantly effective in reducing the severity of acute attacks of migraine.

Isometheptene mucate

Isometheptene is a sympathomimetic, used in the treatment of migraine and throbbing headache for its vasoconstrictor effect. It is included at a dose of 65 mg in combination with paracetamol 325 mg in Midrid capsules (Manx). The dosage is two capsules at once, followed by one every hour if necessary, up to a maximum of five capsules in 12 hours. Midrid is not licensed for use in children or during pregnancy or breastfeeding.

The cautions, contraindications and interactions that apply to this product are described under Sympathomimetics in the chapter on Cough.

A double-blind, randomised, parallel-group trial[2] that compared a combination product containing isometheptene mucate, paracetamol and dichloralphenazone with sumatriptan succinate concluded that both preparations were safe and effective when used early in the treatment of an acute migraine attack, and that the isometheptene preparation may have a slight advantage in the early treatment of mild-to-moderate migraine. The *British National Formulary*, on the other hand, denotes Midrid as a product considered "less suitable for prescribing" and states that other more effective treatments are available.

Prochlorperazine

Prochlorperazine is licensed for nausea and vomiting associated with migraine.

Mode of action and use

Prochlorperazine is a phenothiazine derivative, closely related chemically to antihistamines such as promethazine and antipsychotics such as chlorpromazine and trifluoperazine. Although it has been used as an antipsychotic, it is generally used at lower doses for the treatment of vertigo and the prevention of nausea and vomiting, for which it has a long history of use as a prescription medicine. In 2001, prochlorperazine maleate buccal tablets were licensed as a Pharmacy medicine for the treatment of nausea and vomiting associated with migraine.

Absorption directly into the circulation via the buccal route avoids delay in absorption from the stomach because of the gastric stasis that often accompanies migraine, and first-pass hepatic metabolism. The drug can therefore be supplied at a lower dose than via the oral route. A double-blind trial[3] has compared buccal prochlorperazine 3 mg with oral ergotamine tartarate 1 mg plus caffeine 100 mg and with placebo (buccal or oral) for treatment of acute migraine. The proportion of patients reporting resolution of headache and accompanying symptoms within 2 hours with prochlorperazine was more than double that for the ergotamine preparation or placebo. The prochlorperazine presentation was also found to be easy to use and was well tolerated.

Restrictions and contraindications

The licensing conditions only permit supply if migraine has already been diagnosed by a doctor. Use is restricted to adults of 18 years and over, is contraindicated in pregnancy and in breastfeeding women. It is also contraindicated in patients with impaired hepatic function, narrow-angle glaucoma, prostatic hypertrophy, epilepsy or Parkinson's disease.

Side-effects and interactions

These are typical of phenothiazines and are as described for antihistamines in the chapters on Motion sickness and Cough. Postural hypotension is also possible, particularly in volume-depleted patients. Extrapyramidal side-effects are also a possibility, but are unlikely at the licensed dosage.

Dosage

Buccal tablets are placed in the buccal cavity, high up between the upper lip and gum, and allowed to dissolve there. One or two tablets may be taken twice daily for up to 2 days if necessary.

Product

- Buccastem M
  Reckitt Benckiser

Sumatriptan and zolmitriptan

Mode of action and efficacy

Serotonin (5-hydroxytriptamine, 5HT) is a neurotransmitter and mediator of blood-vessel and smooth-muscle contraction throughout the body. The $5HT_{1D}$ receptor mediates cerebral vasoconstriction.

Triptans are $5HT_{1D}$-receptor agonists; they cause constriction of the cerebral arteries and counteract the cranial vasodilatation that is thought to be responsible for migraine attacks. Triptans are now established as a first-line treatment for migraine.

Sumatriptan was the first triptan to be licensed; it acts rapidly but is poorly absorbed. Zolmitriptan was introduced more recently; it has higher bioavailability than sumatriptan, is more lipophilic and crosses the blood–brain barrier more readily. A Cochrane review[4] has concluded that sumatriptan is an effective drug for the treatment of a single acute attack of migraine, and it is well tolerated, although minor adverse events are not uncommon. The review also states that other triptans are generally similar in terms of efficacy and occurrence of adverse events. Another systematic review[5] and two randomised controlled trials[6,7] found zolmitriptan and sumatriptan to be significantly more effective than placebo in providing headache relief, with no significant difference between them.

Licensing conditions and dosage

Both sumatriptan and zolmitriptan are licensed for acute relief of migraine attacks, with or without aura, in adults aged 18–65 years. Treatment may not be supplied for prophylaxis or for patients who are:

- pregnant or breastfeeding
- have existing medical conditions, including cardiovascular conditions, hypertension, peripheral vascular disease, liver or kidney disorders
- have any neurological condition or symptoms, including epilepsy
- are allergic to either drug
- are taking concurrent medication for migraine
- are assessed as having a high cardiovascular risk, using the factors in the cardiovascular risk prediction charts in the *British National Formulary*.

Dosage

Sumatriptan, one 50 mg tablet, or zolmitriptan, one 2.5 mg orodipsersible tablet, should be taken as soon as possible after onset of an attack. A second dose may be taken after 2 hours if migraine recurs. If there is no response to the first tablet, a second tablet should not be taken for the same attack.

The maximum dosage is two tablets in 24 hours.

Referral

Referral to a doctor should be made if:

- attacks last longer than 24 hours
- attacks become more frequent or symptoms change
- the patient generally has four or more attacks per month
- the patient does not recover completely between attacks
- the patient is over 50 years of age and is suffering a migraine attack for the first time.

Side-effects

Side-effects associated with sumatriptan and zolmitriptan are usually mild and transient. The most common include sensations of tingling, heat, heaviness, pressure or tightness of any part of the body. Flushing, dizziness, feelings of weakness, fatigue, and nausea and vomiting may also be experienced.

Interactions

Sumatriptan and zolmitriptan should be avoided by patients taking selective serotonin-reuptake inhibitors, monoamine oxidase inhibitors, moclobemide, St John's Wort, and other vasoconstrictor migraine treatments, especially ergotamine and methysergide.

Some patients have cross-sensitivity to sumatriptan and sulphonamides; patients who are allergic to sulphonamides should not take sumatriptan.

Product

- Sumatriptan: Imigran Relief 50 mg tablets
  GSK Consumer Healthcare

PRODUCT SELECTION POINTS

- The first-line treatment for migraine recommended by medical authorities is simple analgesics, taken as soon as possible. Soluble formulations may speed absorption and overcome the effects of gastric stasis that is commonly part of the condition.
- Prochloperazine can be used to counteract nausea and vomiting accompanying migraine headache and there is also a combination product containing analgesic components with buclizine as an anti-emetic.
- Triptans are effective but should be held in reserve as second-line treatment in case simple analgesics fail.
- All treatments should be taken at the first indication of an impending attack if there are warning signs, otherwise as soon as the first symptoms are experienced.

PRODUCT RECOMMENDATIONS

- First-line treatment – simple analgesics, with an anti-emetic if necessary.
- Second-line treatment if analgesics fail – sumatriptan or zolmitriptan.

REFERENCES

1. Adam EI. A treatment for the acute migraine attack. *J Int Med Res* 1987; 15: 71–75.
2. Freitag FG, Cady R, DiSerio F, *et al.* Comparative study of a combination of isometheptene mucate, dichloralphenazone with acetaminophen and sumatriptan succinate in the treatment of migraine. *Headache* 2001; 41: 391–398.
3. Sharma S, Prasad A, Nehru R, *et al.* Efficacy and tolerability of prochlor-perazine buccal tablets in treatment of acute migraine. *Headache* 2002; 42: 896–902.
4. McCrory DC, Gray RN. Oral sumatriptan for acute migraine. *The Cochrane Library*, issue 3. Chichester, UK: John Wiley & Sons, 2003 (www.thecochranelibrary.com).
5. Ferrari MD, Goadsby PJ, Roon KI, *et al.* Triptans (serotonin, 5–HT1B/1D agonists) in migraine: detailed results and methods of a meta-analysis of 53 trials. *Cephalalgia* 2002; 22: 633–658.
6. Gruffyd-Jones K, Kies B, Middleton A, *et al.* Zolmitriptan versus suma-triptan for the acute oral treatment of migraine: a randomized, double-blind, international study. *Eur J Neurol* 2001; 8: 237–245.
7. Gallagher R, Dennidh G, Spierings E, *et al.* A comparative trial of zolmitriptan and sumatriptan for the acute oral treatment of migraine. *Headache* 2000; 40: 119–128.

Motion sickness

Motion sickness is a term covering all forms of travel sickness, by any type of transport – air, sea or land.

CAUSES

Motion sickness is a form of vertigo in which autonomic symptoms predominate. It may include, in addition to nausea and vomiting, increased salivation, general malaise, pallor, sweating, yawning and hyperventilation. Gastric motility is reduced and digestion impaired. Two main theories have been put forward to account for motion sickness:

- overstimulation of the vestibular apparatus of the inner ear caused by unaccustomed types of movement
- conflict between stimuli received in the brain from the vestibular system, the eyes and other non-vestibular spatial receptors.

Vomiting is a complex process involving both the central nervous system (CNS) and the gastrointestinal system. It is mediated by the vomiting centre in the medulla of the brain. The vomiting centre receives stimuli from peripheral areas such as the gastric mucosa and from within the CNS. The chemoreceptor trigger zone in the brain operates in close association with the vomiting centre; it is stimulated by many drugs and by certain metabolic disturbances, and it activates the vomiting centre. The vomiting centre is also activated by impulses from the gastrointestinal tract and the vestibular apparatus of the inner ear, the activity of the latter being involved in the causation of motion sickness. Once activated, the vomiting centre transmits stimuli via a cranial nerve to the abdominal musculature, stomach and oesophagus to initiate vomiting.

First-generation antihistamines and hyoscine (scopolamine) are used in non-prescription medicines for the prophylaxis and treatment of motion sickness.

Antihistamines

Compounds available

Compounds available are:

- cinnarizine
- meclozine
- promethazine teoclate and promethazine hydrochloride.

Mode of action, dosage and products

In addition to their anti-allergic, antipruritic, antitussive and antimuscarinic effects, first-generation H_1-antagonists also have, in varying degrees, anti-emetic properties and some are used exclusively for these actions. Their effectiveness for this indication may relate to their antimuscarinic activity, but it has also been proposed that the anti-emetic activity results from blockade of dopamine D_2-receptors in the brain.

Second-generation antihistamines, having much lower lipid solubility than first-generation compounds, do not cross the blood–brain barrier to a significant extent and exert little or no central activity. Tests have shown them to be of no value as hypnotics or as prophylaxis for motion sickness.

The compounds used against motion sickness are selected primarily for their anti-emetic properties, but factors such as duration of action and side-effects are also taken into account. All the compounds listed above are thought to be of similar efficacy, although there appears to be no evidence from comparative trials. All preparations for motion sickness are intended for prophylactic use, and are less effective once nausea or vomiting has begun. Apart from the risk of the drugs being vomited up, they will be absorbed more slowly because gastric motility is decreased.

- **Cinnarizine**

  Cinnarizine is a piperazine derivative, and compounds in this group generally possess anti-emetic properties. Cinnarizine causes some drowsiness, but antimuscarinic side-effects do not appear to be a problem. Peak plasma concentrations occur 2–4 hours after administration, and the half-life is 3–6 hours. A trial[1] found cinnarizine, 25 mg, to be no more effective than placebo in rough seas, although 50 mg was more effective. An open study[2] of cinnarizine for car sickness in children found it to be effective in preventing vomiting and to be highly rated by subjects.

  For adults, a loading dose of 30 mg is recommended 2 hours before the start of a journey, followed by one 15 mg tablet 8-hourly throughout the journey. Half this dose may be given to children aged 5–12 years, but cinnarizine is not licensed for use in younger children.

- **Meclozine**

  Meclozine is a piperazine and is considered to be among the least sedating compounds in this group and to have low antimuscarinic activity. It is long-acting. In a double-blind crossover trial,[3] meclozine was found to be less effective against motion sickness than transdermal hyoscine (scopolamine).

  The adult dose is two 12.5 mg tablets taken the night before or 1 hour before travelling, repeated once every 24 hours if necessary. The dose for children aged 6–12 years is half the adult dose, and for children aged 2–6 years is one-quarter the adult dose.

- **Promethazine teoclate and promethazine hydrochloride**
  Promethazine teoclate and promethazine hydrochloride are phenothiazines. They have marked antimotion sickness activity, but also marked antimuscarinic properties, and sedation is common. Both compounds have been widely used for the treatment of nausea, vomiting and vertigo. The sedative effect of promethazine hydrochloride is sometimes considered to be an advantage in young children on long journeys. (Promethazine hydrochloride has other non-prescription uses: see chapters on Cough, Hay fever and Temporary sleep disturbance.)

  Promethazine teoclate is long acting. The initial dose for adults and child over 10 years of age is one 25 mg tablet, taken 2 hours before a short journey or the night before a long journey, with further 25 mg doses every 24 hours if required. Half the adult dose can be given to children aged 5–10 years.

  Promethazine hydrochloride is also long acting, and is licensed for use in children from the age of 2 years. It has the advantage of being available as tablets in two strengths (10 mg and 25 mg) and as an elixir (5 mg per 5 mL). Dosage schedules are as for promethazine teoclate, but one 10 mg tablet is recommended for 5–10-year-olds, and a 5 mg dose of the elixir (5 mL) for children aged 2–5 years.

Hyoscine hydrobromide

Mode of action and dosage

Hyoscine (scopolamine) hydrobromide is a naturally occurring alkaloid; it competitively inhibits the actions of acetylcholine at the muscarinic receptors of autonomic effector sites innervated by parasympathetic nerves. It has a central as well as a peripheral action, as it is lipid-soluble and crosses the blood–brain barrier.

Hyoscine is probably the most effective drug for prevention of motion sickness,[4] although it is relatively short acting when used orally and has more pronounced antimuscarinic side-effects than antihistamines. A double-blind trial[5] showed that hyoscine was more effective against seasickness than cinnarizine, although the latter was better tolerated in having less marked side-effects. As motion severity increased, comparative tolerability of hyoscine improved.

Hyoscine is available as a transdermal patch and in placebo-controlled trials this formulation was found to be more effective than oral meclozine for prophylaxis of motion sickness.[3]

Doses vary slightly between products, but the *British National Formulary* recommends, for adults, hyoscine hydrobromide 0.3 mg 30 minutes before travelling, followed by 0.3 mg every 6 hours if required, to a maximum of three doses in 24 hours. The recommended dose for children over 10 years of age is 0.15–0.3 mg and for children aged 4–10 years is 75–150 micrograms (0.075–0.15 mg). Kwells Kids (Bayer) and Joy-Rides (GSK Consumer Healthcare) are licensed for use in children from ages 4 and 6 years, respectively. The transdermal patch should be applied to a clean, hairless area of skin behind the ear, 5–6 hours before travelling. It is effective for up to 72 hours.

Antihistamines and hyoscine

Adverse effects, cautions and contraindications

Antihistamines and hyoscine possess peripheral and central antimuscarinic activity and have similar adverse effects, including sedation, dry mouth, blurred vision, urinary retention and constipation. However, these do not normally cause problems at the low doses used over short periods.

Antihistamines and hyoscine should be avoided by patients suffering from glaucoma or prostatic hypertrophy, and in general should be used with caution in the elderly and in patients with epilepsy or cardiac or cardiovascular disease. Paradoxical CNS stimulation may occur with antihistamines in children, resulting in insomnia and excitement and, rarely, nightmares, hallucinations and even convulsions. Photosensitivity reactions have been reported with promethazine. Alcohol should be avoided when taking any preparation for motion sickness.

In pregnancy, use under medical supervision is advised for antihistamine travel-sickness products, because of fears of possible congenital malformations. Antihistamines were at one time routinely prescribed for morning sickness, but concerns arose over a product containing the antihistamine doxylamine and it was withdrawn from the market in 1983. Although no firm causal link was established between this product or other antihistamines and congenital abnormalities,[6] antihistamines have since been used with caution in pregnancy. Similar fears have not been expressed about hyoscine products and no warnings have been issued against their use in pregnancy. However, it is prudent to avoid any medication in pregnancy, if possible, and certainly in the first trimester.

Interactions

Antihistamines and hyoscine interact with other drugs that cause sedation or have antimuscarinic effects, including tricyclic antidepressants, monoamine oxidase inhibitors, phenothiazines, hypnotics, nefopam, amantadine and disopyramide. Dry mouth caused by the antimuscarinic effects of antihistamines and hyoscine may reduce the effect of sublingual nitrates.

Products

- Cinnarizine
  - Stugeron 15 tablets
    McNeil

- Meclozine
  - Sea-legs tablets
    SSL International
  - Traveleeze Soft and Chewy pastilles
    Ernest Jackson

- Promethazine hydrochloride
  — Phenergan tablets (25 mg and 10 mg) and elixir
    Sanofi-Aventis

- Promethazine teoclate
  — Avomine tablets
    Manx

- Hyoscine hydrobromide
  — Joy-rides (0.15 mg)
    GSK Consumer Healthcare
  — Kwells tablets (0.3 mg)
  — Kwells Kids tablets (0.15 mg)
    both *Bayer*
  — Scopoderm 1.5 mg patches
    Novartis Consumer Health

PRODUCT SELECTION POINTS

- All the available products appear to be effective for the prophylaxis of motion sickness, but hyoscine hydrobromide is probably the most effective, especially for sea travel.
- The antimuscarinic side-effects of hyoscine are generally more pronounced than those of the antihistamines.
- Meclozine combines the advantages of relatively few side-effects with prolonged action.
- Promethazine hydrochloride can be used for children from the age of 2 years.

PRODUCT RECOMMENDATIONS

- Adults and older children: for short journeys – hyoscine hydrobromide; for long journeys – meclozine or transdermal hyoscine.
- Children aged 2–5 years – promethazine hydrochloride.

REFERENCES

1. Doweck I, Gordon CR, Spitzer O, *et al.* Effect of cinnarizine in the prevention of seasickness. *Aviat Space Environ Med* 1994; 65: 606–609.
2. Macnair AL. Cinnarizine in the prophylaxis of car sickness in children. *Curr Med Res Opin* 1983; 8: 451–455.
3. Dahl E, Offer-Ohlsen D, Lillevold PE, Sandvik L. Transdermal scopolamine, oral meclizine, and placebo in motion sickness. *Clin Pharmacol Ther* 1984; 36: 116–120.
4. Spinks AB, Wasiak J, Villanueva EV, Bernath V. Scopolamine for preventing and treating motion sickness. *The Cochrane Library,* issue 3. Chichester, UK: John Wiley & Sons, 2004 (www.thecochranelibrary.com).
5. Pingree BJ, Pethybridge RJ. A comparison of the efficacy of cinnarizine with scopolamine in the treatment of seasickness. *Aviat Space Environ Med* 1994; 65: 597–605.
6. Kutcher JS, Engle A, Firth J, Lamm SH. Bendectin and birth defects. II: Ecological analyses. *Birth Defects Res A Clin Mol Teratol* 2003; 67: 88–97.

Mouth ulcers

Mouth ulcers (recurrent aphthous stomatitis) are a common condition of the oral mucosa. Estimates of the proportion of the population affected vary from 5 to 20%. About 75% of cases are minor aphthous ulcers that are self-limiting and can usually be treated without recourse to a doctor.

CAUSES

Aphthous ulcers are painful, shallow ulcers up to 5 mm in diameter, occurring singly or in groups of up to five lesions on the tongue or the mucosal surfaces of the lips and cheeks. They usually appear suddenly, although some patients experience sensitivity and tingling beforehand, and disappear just as abruptly – usually within 7–14 days. Both adults and children can be affected.

Patients who have ulcers that are significantly larger, persist longer or are relatively painless should not be treated but should be referred immediately to a doctor.

The cause of aphthous stomatitis remains unknown, although several causes have been suggested with some degree of justification, including stress, trauma of the oral mucosa, infection, vitamin B or iron deficiency, hormonal changes and heredity, but none has been conclusively proven. Several drugs also appear to induce mouth ulcers. As the cause is unknown, treatment can only be symptomatic; anti-inflammatories (including corticosteroids) seem to be the most effective, but a wide range of products containing local anaesthetics, antiseptics and astringents is also available.

TREATMENT

Corticosteroids

Compounds available

Compounds available are:

- hydrocortisone sodium succinate
- triamcinolone acetonide.

Mode of action

Hydrocortisone is a naturally occurring glucocorticoid secreted by the adrenal cortex. Chemically it is a C21-steroid containing a 17-hydroxy group. Esterification of glucocorticoids at the 17 or 21 positions with fatty acids generally increases topical activity; hydrocortisone sodium succinate is esterified at the 21 position. Fluorination and the formation of cyclic acetonides at the 16 and 17 positions of glucocorticoids, both of which are features of the chemical structure of triamcinolone acetonide, further increase topical anti-inflammatory activity.

Corticosteroids are widely used as topical anti-inflammatory agents. Their action is thought to be exerted through two mechanisms:

- stabilisation of lysosomal membranes, reducing the release of inflammatory lytic enzymes
- inhibition of phospholipase A, which reduces the release of arachidonic acid from phospholipids in cell membranes, with a consequent inhibition of prostaglandin synthesis.

Mouth ulcer tissue is intensely inflamed and corticosteroids would therefore be expected to be helpful. There is weak evidence from randomised controlled trials[1] that topical corticosteroids may reduce the duration and pain of ulcers and hasten pain relief, and that they reduce the number of ulcer days compared with control preparations.

Administration and use

Hydrocortisone sodium succinate is presented as small white pellets. One should be placed in the mouth in close proximity to the ulcer(s) and allowed to dissolve slowly. This can be done four times a day for a maximum of 5 days. Pellets are useful when ulcers are situated between the gum and cheek or beneath the tongue, but may be difficult to maintain in position elsewhere in the mouth.

Triamcinolone acetonide is presented in carmellose (carboxy-methylcellulose) gelatin paste, which is insoluble in saliva and adheres to the oral mucosa to form a thick layer. (Carmellose gelatin paste can be used alone for the mechanical protection of oral lesions.) The preparation is applied to the ulcer with a finger, at bedtime and two or three times a day, up to four times daily for a maximum of 5 days. The area of application should be dry to ensure that the preparation adheres, and some manual dexterity is required to get the paste into areas of difficult access.

Cautions and contraindications

There are no significant side-effects with either product. Both can be used for children and elderly patients with the normal precautions, but should not be used in pregnancy, as high topical doses in experimental animals have caused fetal abnormalities. Patients with a history of hypersensitivity to product components, and those with tuberculous or viral lesions should not use these products. Patients presenting with both mouth ulcers and cold sores or possible bacterial infection should be referred, as concomitant anti-infective treatment might be needed.

Products

- Corlan pellets (hydrocortisone 2.5 mg, as the sodium succinate)
  UCB Pharma

- Adcortyl in Orabase (triamcinolone acetonide 0.1%)
  Bristol-Myers Squibb

Benzydamine hydrochloride

Benzydamine hydrochloride is a non-steroidal anti-inflammatory and analgesic drug, available for the treatment of mouth ulcers as an oral rinse and spray, both of which contain 0.15% benzydamine hydrochloride. The oral rinse has been shown to be effective in the treatment of some oral inflammatory conditions. There is poor evidence of its effectiveness against mouth ulcers, although in two small trials[2,3] it provided some relief of pain. Its principal advantage may be that, as a solution, it can reach areas inaccessible to other mouth ulcer treatments.

For adults, 15 mL rinse should be used every 1.5–3 hours for up to 7 days. If stinging occurs, the solution may be diluted with water. The rinse is not suitable for children under 12 years of age.

Product

- Difflam oral rinse
  3M

Chlorhexidine gluconate

Chlorhexidine gluconate (digluconate) is a bisbiguanide antimicrobial agent, effective against a wide range of bacteria, viruses, fungi and yeasts. Chlorhexidine gluconate mouth rinses have been found to reduce the duration of episodes of aphthous ulceration[1] and to reduce pain. (A trial using 0.1% hexetidine [Oraldene, Pfizer Consumer Healthcare], another bactericidal and fungicidal antiseptic, found it to be no better than placebo in reducing the duration or number of mouth ulcer lesions or pain.[4])

Corsodyl mouthwash contains 0.2% chlorhexidine gluconate. The mouth should be thoroughly rinsed with about 10 mL undiluted solution twice daily. It can be used by children and the elderly, and is considered safe to use during pregnancy and breastfeeding.

Product

- Corsodyl mouthwash
  GSK Consumer Healthcare

Other mouth ulcer treatments

A wide range of products in the form of gels, paints, pastilles and mouthwashes is available, most of which contain combinations of anaesthetic, analgesic, antimicrobial and astringent ingredients. The rationale for the use of these ingredients appears to be similar to that for cold sore products (see chapter on Cold sores).

The inclusion of local anaesthetic and analgesic agents seems reasonable, as they should be useful in reducing pain and discomfort until lesions resolve. Many formulations are, however, aqueous or aqueous–alcoholic liquids or gels which tend to be diluted fairly rapidly and washed away from the site of application by saliva, requiring frequent re-application. The use of pastilles or sore-throat lozenges containing local anaesthetic placed close up against lesions and allowed to dissolve slowly may produce a more prolonged effect. Some lozenges containing higher concentrations of local anaesthetic are unsuitable for children. The Committee on Safety of Medicine's warning against use of aspirin in children does not extend to topical products containing salicylates. However, excessive use of products containing choline salicylate or salicylic acid may lead to ulceration and salicylate poisoning.

There is no evidence that antiseptics or astringents have any effect on mouth ulcers, although the former may help prevent secondary infections.

Product examples

Components are given in parentheses.

- Compound Thymol Glycerin BP 1988

- Anbesol liquid (lidocaine hydrochloride, chlorocresol, cetylpyridinium chloride)
- Anbesol Adult Strength gel (lidocaine 2%)
  both *SSL International*

- Bonjela gel (choline salicylate, cetalkonium chloride)
  Reckitt Benckiser

- Frador paint (menthol, chlorbutanol, prepared storax, benzoin)
  Fenton

- Medijel gel and pastilles (lidocaine hydrochloride, aminoacridine hydrochloride)
  Dendron

- Pyralvex paint (anthraquinone glycosides, salicylic acid)
  Norgine

- Rinstead sugar-free pastilles (menthol, cetylpyridinium chloride)
  Schering-Plough

Several lozenges marketed for sore throat also contain combinations of local anaesthetic and antimicrobial agents and could be used for mouth ulcers.

PRODUCT SELECTION POINTS

- There is some evidence of effectiveness for corticosteroids, benzydamine and chlorhexidine.
- Triamcinolone acetonide in carmellose paste and hydrocortisone pellets are indicated specifically for mouth ulcers.
- Products containing local anaesthetic or analgesic agents should provide symptomatic relief; pastilles or lozenges may have a more prolonged effect than liquids or aqueous gels.

PRODUCT RECOMMENDATIONS

- First choice – triamcinolone acetonide in carmellose paste or hydrocortisone pellets, because they are specifically indicated for mouth ulcers. Benzydamine and chlorhexidine mouthwashes also appear to be effective and may be more suitable for multiple ulcers and ulcers to which it is difficult to apply corticosteroid preparations.
- Second choice – pastilles or lozenges containing local anaesthetic or analgesic constituents.

REFERENCES

1. Porter S, Scully C. Aphthous ulcers (recurrent). Clinical Evidence (www.clinicalevidence.com/ceweb/conditions/orh/1303/1303_I1.jsp#summary) Accessed 16/11/05)
2. Edres MA, Scully C, Gelbier M. Use of proprietary agents to relieve recurrent aphthous stomatitis. *Br Dent J* 1997; 182: 144–146.
3. Matthews RW, Scully CM, Levers BG, Hislop WS. Clinical evaluation of benzydamine, chlorhexidine, and placebo mouthwashes in the management of recurrent aphthous stomatitis. *Oral Surg Oral Med Oral Pathol* 1987; 63: 189–191.
4. Chadwick B, Addy M, Walker DM. Hexetidine mouthrinse in the management of minor aphthous ulceration and as an adjunct to oral hygiene. *Br Dent J* 1991; 171: 83–87.

Nappy rash

Nappy rash is a form of irritant dermatitis.

The causes of nappy rash are not known with certainty, but faecal enzymes and ammonia from urine are likely contributory agents, acting on skin that has become damaged by prolonged exposure to moisture and occlusion under nappies. Further irritants are residual detergents and disinfectants left in cotton nappies after washing. The incidence of nappy rash has decreased with the introduction of disposable nappies that draw urine away from the nappy surface and leave the skin dry.[1,2]

Nappy rash can be complicated by bacterial and fungal infection, and some products for nappy rash contain antiseptics to inhibit bacterial growth and reduce the likelihood of infection. Weeping or crusting of the rash indicates that bacterial infection is present, referral to a doctor thus being necessary. Secondary fungal infection (candidiasis) can be identified by the presence of small, red papules at the edge of the rash, and can be treated without prescription with clotrimazole 1% cream (see chapter on Athlete's foot).

TREATMENT

Hydrocortisone may be used by doctors to treat severe nappy rash, but this option is not available to pharmacists, as topical hydrocortisone is not licensed for non-prescription use in children under 10 years of age.

Over-the-counter treatments for nappy rash are based on soothing and rehydrating damaged skin, providing a physical barrier between the skin and irritant agents, and reducing the possibility of bacterial infection. The main constituents of preparations are emollients, skin protectants, antiseptics and silicone barrier agents. There is considerable variation in the formulas and approach to treatment between preparations marketed for this indication, as a brief review of the most popular products will illustrate.

Product examples

- **Zinc and Castor Oil Ointment BP**

  This has been a popular treatment for several generations. It contains zinc oxide in a greasy emollient base. Zinc oxide is claimed to have antiseptic, astringent, soothing and protective properties. The main effect of this formulation is to provide a hydrophobic and mechanical protective barrier on the skin. Nappies impregnated with zinc oxide incorporated into petroleum jelly have been shown to reduce skin barrier damage and erythema in nappy rash.[3]

- **Conotrane cream**

  Yamanouchi

  This product contains benzalkonium chloride and dimeticone in an emollient cream base. Benzalkonium is one of two antiseptic compounds used in nappy rash preparations, cetrimide being the other. Both are quaternary ammonium surfactant compounds with activity against a wide range of Gram-positive and some Gram-negative bacteria. Their detergent properties are useful in loosening debris and dead tissue from the skin. They do not generally cause irritation and are widely used as skin antiseptics. Dimeticone is a water-repellent fluid silicone, used as a topical barrier to protect skin against water-soluble irritants.

- **Drapolene cream**

  Chefaro UK

  This is an antiseptic and emollient product, containing benzalkonium chloride and cetrimide in a water-miscible cream base.

- **Hewletts cream**

  Kestrel

  This product contains zinc oxide in an emollient cream base.

- **Metanium ointment**
  Roche Consumer Health

  Metanium ointment contains titanium salts, which have an action on the skin similar to zinc oxide, in a silicone-paraffin base. The overall effect is that of a mechanical barrier and occlusive emollient. Titanium salts may stain clothing and bedclothes.

- **Morhulin ointment**
  Thornton & Ross

  This product contains cod liver oil and zinc oxide in an ointment base. Cod liver oil has been claimed to promote wound healing, but the evidence does not support this,[4] and in this preparation it has no special properties beyond its water-resistant and emollient effects.

- **Sudocrem antiseptic healing cream**
  Forest

  Sudocrem contains zinc oxide in an emollient cream base.

Application and practical points

All preparations for nappy rash should be applied after each nappy change until the rash has cleared, and the following advice may be given to reduce future occurrences.

- Change nappies frequently, and promptly after defecation, to minimise contact of moisture and excretion products with the skin.
- Clean the nappy area thoroughly at each nappy change, and dry thoroughly afterwards.
- Nappies should be left off as much as possible, to allow air to circulate and help dry the skin.

- Washable nappies should be rinsed thoroughly after being washed and disinfected, as any residual detergent or bleach can act as an irritant.

PRODUCT SELECTION POINTS

- Preparations for nappy rash are based on emollients – agents that act as physical barriers between the skin and irritants – and antiseptics, individual products containing different combinations of these. Choice is usually based on personal preference.
- A good nappy-changing routine can reduce the occurrence of nappy rash.

PRODUCT RECOMMENDATIONS

- Choice is according to personal preference.
- For nappy rash complicated with candidiasis – clotrimazole 1% cream.

REFERENCES

1. Akin F, Spraker M, Aly R, *et al*. Effects of breathable disposable diapers: reduced prevalence of Candida and common diaper dermatitis. *Pediatr Dermatol* 2001; 18: 282–290.
2. Odio M, Friedlander SF. Diaper dermatitis and advances in diaper technology. *Curr Opin Pediatr* 2000; 12: 342–346.
3. Baldwin S, Odio MR, Haines SL, *et al*. Skin benefits from continuous topical administration of a zinc oxide/petrolatum formulation by a novel disposable diaper. *J Eur Acad Dermatol Venereol* 2001; 15 (Suppl 1): 5–11.
4. Sweetman SC, ed. *Martindale: The complete drug reference,* 34th edn. London: Pharmaceutical Press, 2005; 1425.

Oral thrush

Oral thrush appears as creamy-white patches on the oral mucosa that may be mistaken for milk curds, but they are difficult to remove and, if scraped away, reveal inflamed patches that may bleed.

CAUSES

Oral thrush (oral candidiasis) is an infection caused by a yeast-like fungus, *Candida albicans*, the same organism that causes vaginal candidiasis and may complicate nappy rash. It is common in newborn babies because they can pick up the organism during passage through an infected birth canal.

Oral thrush can also be contracted by users of inhaled corticosteroids or following antibiotic treatment; such patients should be referred, as infection may indicate reduced immune status. Oral candidiasis can also be a problem in patients with dentures (this condition is called denture stomatitis); such patients should also be referred.

TREATMENT

The standard treatment for infants is miconazole oral gel, which has been shown to be effective[1] and can be recommended by pharmacists. Adults may be referred back from the doctor to the pharmacist for treatment, as the product costs less than a prescription charge. Only the 15 g pack is classified as a Pharmacy medicine; the 80 g pack is a Prescription-only medicine.

Mode of action

See chapter on Athlete's foot.

Dosage and administration

- For babies (from birth) and children up to 6 years of age – apply a small amount of the gel to the affected area with a clean finger twice daily
- For children from 6 years of age and adults – apply four times daily.

The gel should be retained in the mouth for as long as possible.

Interactions and contraindications

Miconazole gel is absorbed from the oral mucosa and at least part of a dose will be swallowed and absorbed systemically. Miconazole potentiates the activity of anticoagulants, antiepileptics and hypoglycaemic drugs. Pharmacists should consult with the doctor if patients are receiving any of the above drugs.

Miconazole has been shown to be fetotoxic, although not teratogenic, in animal studies, and the oral gel is not licensed for use in pregnant women without prescription.

Product

There is only one product:

- Daktarin oral gel (24 mg/mL)
  McNeil

REFERENCE

1. Hoppe JE. Treatment of oropharyngeal candidiasis in immunocompetent infants: a randomized multicenter study of miconazole gel vs. nystatin suspension. The Antifungals Study Group. *Pediatr Infect Dis J* 1997; 16: 288–293.

Pain

(continued . . .)

(continued . . .)

Pain can be treated with non-prescription oral and topical analgesics.

Oral analgesics are based on three compounds – aspirin, ibuprofen and paracetamol. Aspirin and ibuprofen are non-steroidal anti-inflammatory drugs (NSAIDs), have similar pharmacologies and will be considered together. Paracetamol is not an NSAID. All three analgesics are used to treat a wide variety of aches and pains, including headache, migraine, toothache, dysmenorrhoea and muscular and rheumatic pain. They also have antipyretic activity and can be used to alleviate cold and influenza symptoms. One compound may be more suitable than another for particular indications and situations, depending on its mode of action, side-effect profile, etc.

Topical analgesics are applied externally to relieve a variety of painful conditions. A wide range of preparations is available, including NSAIDs, rubefacients and local anaesthetics as the main constituents.

TREATMENT WITH ASPIRIN AND IBUPROFEN

Mode of action

NSAIDs exert their therapeutic action by blocking the enzyme cyclo-oxygenase, thereby preventing the formation of prostaglandins from arachidonic acid, which are produced when tissue is damaged and are major contributors to inflammation and pain. The action of NSAIDs is therefore local at the site of tissue damage, in contrast to the central effect of opioids, which influence the recognition of pain within the brain.

Products formed from arachidonic acid also have a role in platelet aggregation. Aspirin interferes with their synthesis, producing a net anticoagulant effect by inhibiting platelet aggregation. In large doses, aspirin also competitively inhibits vitamin K in the synthesis of clotting factors. Ibuprofen has much less antiplatelet activity.

NSAIDs also inhibit production of cytoprotective prostaglandins in the gastric mucosa, which accounts in part for their tendency to cause gastrointestinal irritation, although the incidence is much lower with ibuprofen than aspirin. Prostaglandin inhibition also explains the antipyretic activity of ibuprofen and aspirin, as prostaglandins are released in the brain during fever and have a potent pyrogenic effect on the temperature-regulating region of the hypothalamus.

Uses

Both aspirin and ibuprofen are licensed for treatment of mild and moderate pain from a wide variety of causes, including dental and musculoskeletal pain and dysmenorrhoea, where their anti-inflammatory activity is particularly useful (see below), and as antipyretics.

Side-effects, cautions and contraindications

Aspirin and ibuprofen have similar side-effects, although these are generally less pronounced with ibuprofen. The most common side-effects are gastric irritation and bleeding. These are more severe with aspirin, which has a direct effect on the gastric mucosa (leading to back-diffusion of acid from the gastric lumen to mucosal tissue), as well as its effect on gastric prostaglandin synthesis. Both drugs should be avoided by patients with ulcers or a history of gastric problems. Minor gastric side-effects can be reduced by taking the drugs with or after food.

Hypersensitivity reactions to aspirin are much more likely to occur in patients with asthma or allergic problems than in the normal population. One in ten patients with asthma may be hypersensitive and suffer severe bronchospasm. Other reactions are urticaria, angioedema and rhinitis. The incidence of hypersensitivity to ibuprofen is much lower, but the drug should be avoided by patients with asthma and anyone who is sensitive to aspirin, unless they have taken ibuprofen before without problems.

Aspirin and ibuprofen should not be recommended to patients with renal, cardiac or hepatic disease, as, like all NSAIDs, they may impair both liver and kidney function. As renal function tends to decline with age, and also because the elderly tend to be particularly vulnerable to gastric side-effects, aspirin and ibuprofen should be used with caution in elderly patients.

Aspirin and ibuprofen should be avoided in the third trimester of pregnancy, as they may delay the onset of labour and have adverse effects on late-stage development in the fetus. Aspirin also increases the risk of haemorrhage during labour. There have been some reports of toxicity during the early stages of pregnancy in animal studies with NSAIDs, so it may be prudent not to recommend the use of aspirin or ibuprofen at all during pregnancy.

Aspirin has been associated with Reye's syndrome, a rare but potentially fatal encephalopathy of infants and children. Aspirin is no longer licensed for use in children under 16 years. Breastfeeding mothers should therefore also avoid aspirin. There is no evidence of an association between ibuprofen and Reye's syndrome.

Interactions

Aspirin potentiates the anticoagulant effect of warfarin because of its inhibitory effect on platelet aggregation and inhibition of vitamin K synthesis. A daily dose of only 600 mg can significantly increase blood clotting time, so patients on anticoagulant therapy must avoid over-the-counter (OTC) aspirin products.

Low doses of aspirin are sometimes prescribed in conjunction with warfarin intentionally, particularly to prevent thrombus formation on prosthetic heart valves; this is safe, provided that prothrombin time is monitored regularly.

Aspirin also reduces excretion of methotrexate, and can cause life-threatening rises in serum levels of the drug. All NSAIDs interfere with renal prostaglandin production, inhibiting perfusion and clearance of methotrexate by the kidney; concurrent administration of ibuprofen should therefore also be avoided.

Ibuprofen reduces the excretion of lithium and can raise plasma concentrations to toxic levels. The drug may also antagonise the diuretic and antihypertensive effects of diuretics, and should not be recommended to patients taking these drugs.

Dosage

- **Aspirin:** adults and children over 16 years of age, 300–900 mg every 4–6 hours when required; maximum daily dose 3600 mg.
- **Ibuprofen**
    - **Infants:** 6–12 months of age, 50 mg three or four times in 24 hours.
    - **Children:** 1–3 years of age, 100 mg; 4–6 years of age, 150 mg; 7–9 years of age, 200 mg; 10–12 years of age, 300 mg. (All doses are to a maximum of three times in 24 hours.)
    - **Adults and children over 12:** 200–400 mg every 4 hours, up to a maximum of 1200 mg daily. (Children's doses can be given accurately using ibuprofen suspension – see below.)

Formulation factors

Aspirin is a weak acid, and peak plasma concentrations are achieved 1–2 hours after administration. Ionisation can be increased by formulation with alkaline salts, speeding up absorption and reducing gastrointestinal side-effects. Some effervescent preparations (e.g. Alka-Seltzer [Bayer]) use sodium bicarbonate as a buffer, but the amounts required are high and use may be inadvisable in patients with high blood pressure or who are taking antihypertensive medication. Calcium carbonate, which does not present this problem, is used in Soluble Aspirin Tablets BP and in Disprin (Reckitt Benckiser). Soluble formulations of ibuprofen are also available. Soluble preparations are useful in the treatment of migraine, as the rate of gastric emptying slows in this condition, delaying absorption and increasing the possibility of gastrointestinal side-effects.

Another method of increasing absorption is to render the drug dispersible by formulating with an amino acid. Nurofen Advance (Crookes) contains ibuprofen lysine, which the manufacturer claims reaches peak plasma levels nearly three times faster than ibuprofen. Disprin Direct (Reckitt Benckiser) contains aspirin with glycine.

Enteric coating has been suggested as a solution to the problem of gastric irritation, and absorption of aspirin from the lower gastro-intestinal tract is efficient. However, there is a delay in absorption while the tablet passes through the stomach, and gastric irritation by aspirin has been shown to be the result of both systemic and local effects. This formulation may be useful for patients taking aspirin regularly as an anti-inflammatory, but its slow onset of action makes it unsuitable for general analgesic OTC indications. (The pack-size restrictions on aspirin introduced in 1998 mean that there is no presentation of enteric-coated aspirin tablets 300 mg licensed for sale without prescription.)

Product examples

Aspirin

- Aspirin Tablets BP

- Alka Rapid Crystals
- Aspro Clear tablets
  both *Bayer*

- Disprin soluble tablets
  Reckitt Benckiser

Ibuprofen

- Ibuprofen 200 mg and 400 mg tablets (non-proprietary)

- Advil tablets (200 mg)
  Wyeth

- Cuprofen tablets (200 mg)
  SSL International

- Librofem (200 mg tablets)
  LPC

- Nurofen (200 mg tablets)
- Nurofen Back Pain SR capsules (300 mg sustained release)
- Nurofen Tension Headache (200 mg ibuprofen lysine tablets)
- Nurofen for Children suspension (licensed for use in babies and children from 6 months of age)
  all *Crookes*

- Relcofen 200 mg and Relcofen 400 mg tablets
  Alpharma

TREATMENT WITH PARACETAMOL

Mode of action

Paracetamol, unlike aspirin and ibuprofen, is not an NSAID. The mechanism of action of paracetamol is not well understood. It has little anti-inflammatory activity but is an effective analgesic and antipyretic. It is postulated that it may selectively inhibit cyclo-oxygenase in the central nervous system rather than in peripheral tissues. However, there is evidence that paracetamol also acts peripherally at pain chemoreceptors.

Side-effects and cautions

Paracetamol is a very safe drug at normal therapeutic dosages, and its only major drawback is hepatotoxicity in overdose. Paracetamol is metabolised in the liver, where it is converted to a highly reactive toxic intermediate, which is normally detoxified by conjugation with glutathione. In overdose, this detoxification mechanism is overwhelmed.

The free toxic metabolite then combines with hepatic macromolecules, causing hepatitis and necrosis, which often prove fatal.

Paracetamol poisoning is particularly dangerous, as the toxic level may not be greatly above the therapeutic level, and symptoms of overdose may not appear for 2 days or more. This allows unwitting overdosage to be continued, and there have been fatalities in patients who were taking large doses, or two or more preparations containing paracetamol, for a minor ailment such as a cold. It is therefore extremely important to ensure that patients do not exceed the recommended dosage and do not use more than one paracetamol-containing product at a time.

Methionine is an effective antidote for paracetamol poisoning if used early enough; one proprietary product (Paradote tablets [Sinclair]) contains paracetamol co-formulated with methionine. It may be considered for situations in which overdosage may occur.

Dosage

- **Adults:** 0.5–1 g every 4–6 hours, to a maximum of 4 g daily.
- **Children:** 3–12 months of age, 60–120 mg; 1–5 years of age, 120–250 mg; 6–12 years of age, 250–500 mg; all 4–6-hourly when necessary, to a maximum of four doses in 24 hours.

Product examples

- Paracetamol Tablets BP

- Alvedon suppositories (60 mg, 125 mg, 250 mg: high price may deter potential purchasers)
  AstraZeneca

- Calpol infant suspension
- Calpol 6 Plus suspension
  both *Pfizer Consumer Healthcare*

- Disprol Soluble paracetamol tablets (120 mg)
  Reckitt Benckiser

- Fenpaed suspension and sachets
  Pinewood

- Hedex tablets
  GSK Consumer Healthcare

- Infadrops (100 mg/mL)
  Goldshield Healthcare

- Panadol tablets
  GSK Consumer Healthcare

- Paracets capsules
  Sussex Pharmaceuticals

Restriction of pack sizes

In order to reduce the incidence of poisoning incidents with aspirin and paracetamol, in 1998 the Government introduced legislation to reduce pack sizes and the total quantity of these drugs that could be supplied. The maximum pack size of non-effervescent aspirin or paracetamol tablets or capsules available from pharmacies is now 32; a total of three packs can be sold at the discretion of the pharmacist. In other outlets the maximum pack size is 16, although there is no restriction on the number of packs that can be supplied.

The maximum pack sizes of soluble and effervescent formulations for General sale list (GSL) were restricted from September 2005, as follows:

- **Aspirin:** 30 effervescent tablets of maximum strength 325 mg; 20 effervescent tablets of maximum strength 500 mg; 10 sachets of powder or granules.

- **Paracetamol:** effervescent formulations up to a maximum pack size of 30; in packs greater than 30, it remains GSL, but may only be supplied from pharmacies; there is no maximum amount that may be supplied at one time, regardless of pack size.

Evidence of effectiveness of aspirin, ibuprofen and paracetamol

General use for non-prescription analgesia

A review[1] has stated that low-dose ibuprofen is as effective as aspirin and paracetamol for the indications normally treated with OTC medications and is associated with the lowest risk of gastrointestinal toxicity of any NSAIDs. It has also stated that paracetamol is well tolerated and effective in treating mild-to-moderate pain.

Headache

A comparison[2] found that aspirin 650 mg and paracetamol 1000 mg were equally effective for episodic tension headache and that both were significantly more effective than placebo. A comparative trial[3] of ibuprofen 400 mg against paracetamol 1000 mg concluded that both are efficacious analgesic agents for muscle-contraction headache, and that ibuprofen is significantly more effective than paracetamol at these doses. A trial[4] comparing ibuprofen 200 mg with aspirin 500 mg found that ibuprofen was at least equivalent to aspirin and superior to placebo.

Dental pain

Ibuprofen at a dose of 400 mg has been found to be more effective for dental pain than equivalent doses of aspirin or paracetamol.[5]

Dysmenorrhoea

A Cochrane Review[6] has concluded that NSAIDs are effective in the treatment of primary dysmenorrhoea. Another systematic review[7] concluded that NSAIDs, including aspirin, are all effective and that ibuprofen appeared to have the best risk–benefit ratio. Paracetamol appeared to be less effective than NSAIDs.

Back pain and muscular pain

A systematic review[8] of NSAIDs for the treatment of low-back pain concluded that NSAIDs are effective for short-term symptomatic relief in patients with acute low-back pain, although no specific drug was clearly more effective than others. There was conflicting evidence that NSAIDs were more effective than paracetamol for acute low-back pain. An earlier review[9] concluded that NSAIDs might be effective for short-term symptomatic relief in patients with uncomplicated low-back pain, but are less effective or ineffective in patients with low-back pain with sciatica and patients with sciatica with nerve root symptoms. A comparison of ibuprofen, aspirin and placebo in the treatment of musculoskeletal pain found that ibuprofen was significantly superior to the other two.[10]

Pain and fever in children

A comparison of ibuprofen and paracetamol for fever in children[11] concluded that both are effective antipyretics and both are well tolerated. Ibuprofen appears to have a longer duration of action and is more effective than paracetamol 4–6 hours after administration, which may make it preferable in some circumstances. A meta-analysis of randomised controlled trials[12] concluded that paracetamol and ibuprofen are similar in terms of short-term safety and relief of moderate-to-severe pain in children, but that ibuprofen reduces fever more effectively than paracetamol.

TREATMENT WITH COMBINATION PRODUCTS

The majority of proprietary oral analgesics are not simple formulations of aspirin, ibuprofen or paracetamol but are combination products containing these. The theory behind combination products is that they will be more effective than one drug used alone, and that the dose of each drug can be reduced, thus reducing the possibility of adverse effects. Pain relief is only modestly increased by raising the dose of aspirin and paracetamol so it is postulated that the effect may be increased by including another analgesic, especially if it has a different mechanism of action. Further additional components are sometimes added to treat symptoms associated with the pain. Leading medical opinion (e.g. as represented in the *British National Formulary*) does not generally favour combined analgesics, claiming that low doses of additional ingredients may reduce the severity but increase the range of side-effects without producing significant extra pain relief. Some products (e.g. Anadin Extra [Wyeth] and Disprin Extra [Reckitt Benckiser]) are combinations of aspirin and paracetamol, but the main additional analgesic ingredient used is codeine.

Codeine as additional ingredient

Codeine may be combined with aspirin, paracetamol, aspirin and paracetamol, or ibuprofen. Codeine is a member of the opioid group of analgesics that act directly on opiate receptors in the brain, producing analgesia, respiratory depression, euphoria and sedation. It is a weak narcotic analgesic, useful for the treatment of mild-to-moderate pain. Its major side-effect at non-prescription dosages is constipation.

The combination of codeine with one of the other OTC analgesics is logical from the point of view that they have different mechanisms of action. However, it is argued that, at the dosages at which it codeine is normally included (8 mg per tablet with a two-tablet maximum dose), there is no significant added analgesic efficacy. In addition, several of the indications given by manufacturers for these combinations, such as dysmenorrhoea and dental and rheumatic pain, are not opioid-sensitive. Systematic reviews and meta-analyses[13,14] have concluded that codeine in combination products adds little or nothing to analgesic efficacy. Some newer products contain higher doses of codeine. Dihydrocodeine, which is about as effective as codeine, is combined with paracetamol in one product.

Product examples

- Aspirin and codeine
  - — Co-codaprin tablets and soluble tablets
  - — Codis 500 soluble tablets
    Reckitt Benckiser

- Paracetamol and codeine
  - — Co-codamol tablets and soluble tablets
  - — Paracodol capsules and soluble tablets
    Bayer
  - — Solpadeine Max tablets
    GSK Consumer Healthcare

- Ibuprofen and codeine
  - — Nurofen Plus tablets
    Crookes

- Containing higher dose of codeine
  - — Nurofen Plus (12.5 mg/tablet)
    Crookes
  - — Panadol Ultra (12.8 mg/tablet)
    GSK Consumer Healthcare
  - — Solpadeine Max tablets (12.8 mg/ tablet)
    GSK Consumer Healthcare
  - — Solpaflex tablets (12.8 mg/tablet)
    GSK Consumer Healthcare

- Paracetamol and dihydrocodeine
  - — Paramol tablets (7.5 mg dihydrocodeine per tablet)
    Seton
  - — Co-dydramol tablets (non-proprietary) contain 10 mg dihydrocodeine per tablet and are Prescription-only medicines.

Aloxiprin as additional ingredient

Aloxiprin, a polymeric condensation product of aspirin and aluminium oxide, is co-formulated with aspirin in one product (Askit Powders [Askit]). It is less liable to cause gastric irritation than aspirin, as it is mainly hydrolysed and absorbed in the duodenum, but its is absorbed more slowly and included at such a low dose as to make its contribution doubtful.

Caffeine as additional ingredient

A large number of OTC analgesics contain caffeine, the rationale being that, as a central nervous system stimulant, it will alleviate the depression often associated with pain. However, most preparations contain less caffeine than would be obtained from a cup of tea and half of that from a cup of coffee. In addition, caffeine can add to gastrointestinal adverse effects, is habit forming and may itself induce headache in large doses or on withdrawal.

The value of caffeine in OTC compound analgesic products is disputed. Some trials[13,14] have shown proprietary products to be more effective than single analgesics, while some systematic reviews and meta-analyses[15,16] have concluded that they add little or nothing to efficacy.

Product examples

- Anadin, Anadin Extra, Anadin Extra soluble tablets
  Wyeth

- Propain and Propain Plus caplets
  Ceuta

- Solpadeine Plus capsules, tablets and soluble tablets
  GSK Consumer Healthcare

Antihistamines as additional ingredients

Doxylamine is included at a very low dose with paracetamol, codeine and caffeine in Syndol tablets (SSL International), promoted for tension headache. It is claimed to have muscle-relaxant and sedative effects. In a controlled clinical trial,[17] doxylamine in combination with paracetamol was found to be more effective than the analgesic alone.

Diphenhydramine is included at a low dose in Propain tablets (Ceuta).

PRODUCT SELECTION POINTS FOR ORAL ANALGESICS

- The selection of appropriate non-prescription analgesics is complicated by the fact that the perception of pain is highly subjective and the choice of drug often depends on personal preference.
- The three principal compounds – aspirin, ibuprofen and paracetamol – are all effective for mild-to-moderate pain, although theoretically the first two are better where pain is caused by local inflammation, such as musculoskeletal or dental or dysmenorrhoea.
- Aspirin and ibuprofen have similar indications, but ibuprofen appears to be more effective with fewer adverse and side-effects.
- Paracetamol is a good alternative in situations where aspirin and ibuprofen should be avoided. It is therefore safe for the elderly, children under 16 years of age and pregnant women, and patients with a history of asthma or gastrointestinal problems.
- Aspirin must be avoided by patients taking warfarin or methotrexate, and ibuprofen by those taking lithium. Patients with cardiovascular problems should also avoid ibuprofen.
- It may be wise for patients taking medicines liable to interactions to avoid both aspirin and ibuprofen, given the possibility of cross-sensitivity between NSAIDs.
- Soluble formulations have the advantage of faster action and, in the case of aspirin, reduced gastric irritation. They are

particularly useful in migraine as gastric emptying is slowed during attacks, delaying absorption of the analgesic.

- Combination products containing codeine are worth trying when single-ingredient products are not effective. Constipation is a possible side-effect.
- Additional constituents are included in some analgesic products but at doses too low to be expected to exert an effect.

PRODUCT RECOMMENDATIONS FOR ORAL ANALGESICS

- Ask the patient: they will often know what works for them, even though their choice may not accord with what may be best in theory.
- If asked for a recommendation, the first choice is ibuprofen; paracetamol is recommended for patients in whom ibuprofen is contraindicated.
- If a single analgesic product is not effective, it is worth trying a combination product containing ibuprofen or paracetamol with codeine.

TREATMENT WITH TOPICAL ANALGESICS

Products in this group are applied externally to relieve a variety of painful conditions, including muscular and rheumatic pain, fibrositis, sciatica, lumbago, sprains, strains, bruises, etc.

Non-steroidal anti-inflammatory drugs

Compounds available

Compounds available are:

- benzydamine
- diclofenac
- felbinac
- ibuprofen
- ketoprofen
- piroxicam
- salicylic acid.

Mode of action

The mode of action of NSAIDs is as described above, under ibuprofen and aspirin. Topical NSAIDs are recommended on the premise that the drug acts directly at the affected site, thereby avoiding the systemic adverse effects and side-effects that can result from oral administration. This depends on the drug being absorbed sufficiently into local tissue to exert an effect but without entering the systemic circulation. The skin presents a barrier to absorption and only a small proportion penetrates (4–25% in tests conducted on ibuprofen, depending on the formulation).[18] Once absorbed, NSAIDs show a strong affinity for tissues, although there is evidence that they may be absorbed systemically first and then into the target tissue.

Systematic reviews[19,20] have found topical NSAIDs to be effective over short periods (up to 2 weeks) for chronic muscular conditions and osteoarthritis, and they would therefore appear to be suitable for the kind of acute conditions for which they are licensed for non-prescription sale. In limited studies,[21] topical NSAIDs were found to be as effective as oral NSAIDs for sprains and strains, with a very low incidence of adverse effects. Ketoprofen was significantly better than all other topical NSAIDs.

Uses

Topical NSAIDs are licensed for the treatment of backache, rheumatic and muscular pain, sprains and strains, including sports injuries, and for pain relief in non-serious arthritic conditions.

Side-effects, cautions and contraindications

Topical NSAIDs are generally well tolerated; occasional local reactions have been reported, but these resolve on withdrawal of treatment. Products should not be applied to broken skin, lips or near the eyes. Hands should be washed after application. Topical NSAIDs should not be used with occlusive dressings.

The systemic side-effects associated with oral NSAIDs can occur with topical agents; the risk is increased with application of large amounts. Topical NSAIDs (except benzydamine) are contraindicated in patients who are sensitive to aspirin and other NSAIDs. They are not recommended for use by pregnant or breastfeeding women, or for children under 14 years of age.

Interactions

Serum levels of NSAIDs after topical administration are low, and clinically significant drug interactions are unlikely.

Dosage

- Creams and gels – a 3–10 cm ribbon is applied in a thin layer and massaged in, up to three times a day.
- Sprays – 1–2 mL (5–10 sprays) three or four times a day.

Product examples

Benzydamine
- Difflam cream
  3M

Felbinac
- Traxam pain relief gel
  Goldshield Healthcare

Ibuprofen

At least 12 brands and about 20 variants are available. Two strengths are available: 5%, which may be licensed as GSL, and 10%, which is a Pharmacy medicine.

- Ibuleve gel, mousse, spray and sports gel (5% ibuprofen)
- Ibuleve Maximum Strength gel (10% ibuprofen)
  both *Dendron*

- Mentholatum ibuprofen gel (5% ibuprofen)
  Mentholatum

- Nurofen Gel Maximum Strength (10% ibuprofen)
  Crookes

- Proflex pain relief cream (5% ibuprofen)
  Novartis Consumer Health

Ketoprofen
- Oruvail gel
  Sanofi-Aventis

Piroxicam
- Feldene P gel
  Pfizer Consumer Healthcare

Salicylic acid
- Movelat Relief gel and cream (also contains heparinoid which is said to help disperse oedema from damaged tissue)
  Sankyo

Rubefacients (counterirritants)

Mode of action

Rubefacients are compounds that produce local vasodilation and create a sensation of warmth, exerting an analgesic effect by masking the perception of pain. Massaging greatly enhances this effect by increasing the penetration of the rubefacient into the skin and by stimulating nerve fibres that feed back messages to the brain, over-riding painful stimuli. The pressure exerted also helps to disperse local tissue pain mediators. Massaging is therefore an important component of the action of topical analgesics, including NSAIDs. A systematic review[22] of rubefacients containing salicylate and nicotinate esters concluded, from the best assessment of limited information, that rubefacients containing salicylates may be efficacious in acute pain and moderately to poorly efficacious in chronic arthritic and rheumatic pain. Placebo response rate to rubefacients was, perhaps surprisingly, not high.

Most proprietary rubefacient preparations are mixtures of several ingredients, including salicylates, nicotinates and counterirritant substances from natural sources.

Salicylates

Methyl salicylate, diethylamine salicylate and glycol salicylate are ingredients of many topical analgesic products. As well as being counterirritants, they are hydrolysed in the skin to salicylic acid and have an anti-inflammatory action. Products containing salicylates should therefore be avoided by people who are sensitive to aspirin.

Product examples are:

• Algesal cream
  Thornton & Ross

• Deep Heat Maximum Strength cream
  Mentholatum

- Radian-B Muscle Lotion and Pain Relief spray
  Ransom

- Ralgex Heat spray
  SSL International

Nicotinates

Nicotinates are other popular components of topical analgesics, producing vasodilatation and raised skin temperature.
Product examples are:

- PR Heat spray
  Crookes

- Transvasin Heat Rub
  Thornton & Ross

Capsicum

Capsicum oleoresin and capsaicin, which is obtained from it, are included in several topical analgesics and produce a burning sensation on the skin, which is not accompanied by vasodilatation. Capsaicin works directly on nerve endings, depleting them of substance P, a pain-inducing peptide. A systematic review[23] found that preparations containing 0.025% capsaicin were significantly superior to placebo for musculoskeletal pain, although the number needed to treat (NNT) was quite high (8.1, i.e. for around every eight patients treated one would experience a 50% reduction in pain who would not have done so using placebo).

Product examples are:

- Fiery Jack ointment and cream
  Ransom

- Ralgex cream
  SSL International

Other constituents

Other rubefacient ingredients of analgesic preparations include turpentine oil, camphor and menthol. The last produces a sensation of coolness rather than warmth.

Product examples are:

- Balmosa cream
  Pharmax

- Deep Freeze Cold Gel
  Mentholatum

- Quool patch
  Allmi-Care

- Tiger Balm
  SSL International

Local anaesthetics

Local anaesthetics prevent pain by reversibly blocking conduction along nerve fibres. They are not normally used for the treatment of inflammatory pain. Ointments and gels are sometimes used to ease pain associated with defecation in cases of haemorrhoids and anal fissure.

One product is available:

- Nupercainal ointment (1.1% cinchocaine hydrochloride)
  LPC

Freeze sprays

Freeze sprays contain pressurised liquids that evaporate at low temperature when sprayed onto the skin, producing a loss of sensation until the nerve endings warm up again. They are most useful for treating the sharp, but short-lived, pain caused by minor knocks and sports injuries.

One product is available:

- Ralgex Freeze Spray
  SSL International

Cautions for topical analgesics

All topical analgesic products should be kept well away from the eyes, mouth and mucous membranes, and should not be applied to broken skin. The hands should always be washed after use. Topical analgesics should not be used on young children, whose skin is more sensitive than adults' and in whom reactions are therefore more likely.

PRODUCT SELECTION POINTS FOR TOPICAL ANALGESICS

- All classes of topical analgesics have been shown to be effective for short-term treatment of musculoskeletal pain.
- NSAIDs have the best evidence of efficacy and the lowest NNT.
- Topical NSAID can produce the same adverse and side-effects as oral NSAIDs in sensitive individuals. They should not be used by people sensitive to aspirin and other NSAIDs. Rubefacients containing salicylates are also contraindicated.

- Topical NSAID analgesics are unlikely to interact with other drugs.
- The action of massaging contributes significantly to the effectiveness of topical analgesics.

PRODUCT RECOMMENDATIONS FOR TOPICAL ANALGESICS

Either NSAIDs, which are about as effective as oral NSAIDs, or rubefacients, which are generally cheaper than NSAID preparations.

REFERENCES

1. Moore N. Forty years of ibuprofen use. *Int J Clin Pract Suppl* 2003; 135: 28–31.
2. Peters BH, Fraim CJ, Masel BE. Comparison of 650 mg aspirin and 1,000 mg acetaminophen with each other, and with placebo in moderately severe headache. *Am J Med* 1983; 74: 36–42.
3. Schachtel BP, Furey SA, Thoden WR. Nonprescription ibuprofen and acetaminophen in the treatment of tension-type headache. *J Clin Pharmacol* 1996; 36: 1120–1125.
4. Nebe J, Heier M, Diener HC. Low-dose ibuprofen in self-medication of mild to moderate headache: a comparison with acetylsalicylic acid and placebo. *Cephalalgia* 1995; 15: 531–535.
5. Beaver WT. Review of the analgesic efficacy of ibuprofen. *Int J Clin Pract Suppl* 2003; 135: 13–17.
6. Marjoribanks J, Proctor ML, Farquhar C. Nonsteroidal anti-inflammatory drugs for primary dysmenorrhoea. *The Cochrane Library*, issue 4. Chichester, UK: John Wiley & Sons, 2003 (www.thecochranelibrary.com).
7. Zhang WY, Li Wan Po A. Efficacy of minor analgesics in primary dysmenorrhoea: a systematic review. *Br J Obstet Gynaecol* 1998; 105: 780–789.
8. van Tulder MW, Scholten RJ, Koes BW, Deyo RA. Nonsteroidal anti-inflammatory drugs for low back pain: a systematic review within the framework of the Cochrane Collaboration Back Review Group. *Spine* 2000; 25: 2501–2513.
9. Koes BW, Scholten RJ, Mens JM, Bouter LM. Efficacy of non-steroidal anti-inflammatory drugs for low back pain: a systematic review of randomised clinical trials. *Ann Rheum Dis* 1997; 56: 214–223.
10. Silberman HM. Multiple-dose comparison of suprofen, aspirin, and placebo in the treatment of musculoskeletal pain. *Pharmacology* 1983; 27 (Suppl 1): 65–73.

11. Purssell E. Treating fever in children: paracetamol or ibuprofen? *Br J Comm Nurs* 2002; 7: 316–320.

12. Perrott DA, Piira T, Goodenough B, *et al.* Efficacy and safety of acetaminophen vs ibuprofen for treating children's pain or fever: a meta-analysis. *Arch Pediatr Adolesc Med* 2004; 158: 521–526.

13. Migliardi JR, Armellino JJ, Friedman M, *et al.* Caffeine as an analgesic adjuvant in tension headache. *Clin Pharmacol Ther* 1994 56: 576–586.

14. Diener HC, Pfaffenrath V, Pageler L, *et al.* The fixed combination of acetylsalicylic acid, paracetamol and caffeine is more effective than single substances and dual combination for the treatment of headache: a multicentre, randomized, double-blind, single-dose, placebo-controlled parallel group study. *Cephalalgia* 2005; 25: 776–787.

15. Po AL, Zhang WY. Analgesic efficacy of ibuprofen alone and in combination with codeine or caffeine in post-surgical pain: a meta-analysis. *Eur J Clin Pharmacol* 1998; 53: 303–311.

16. Zhang WY, Po AL. Do codeine and caffeine enhance the analgesic effect of aspirin? A systematic overview. *J Clin Pharm Ther* 1997; 22: 79–97.

17. Gawel MJ, Szalai JF, Stiglick A, *et al.* Evaluation of analgesic agents in recurring headache compared with other clinical pain models. *Clin Pharmacol Ther* 1990; 47: 504–508.

18. Hadgraft J, Whitefield M, Rosher PH. Skin penetration of topical formulations of ibuprofen 5%: an in vitro comparative study. *Skin Pharmacol Appl Skin Physiol* 2003; 16: 137–142.

19. Mason L, Moore RA, Edwards JE, *et al.* Topical NSAIDs for chronic musculoskeletal pain: systematic review and meta-analysis. *BMC Musculoskelet Disord* 2004; 19; 28–35.

20. Lin J, Zhang W, Jones A, Doherty M. Efficacy of topical non-steroidal anti-inflammatory drugs in the treatment of osteoarthritis: meta-analysis of randomised controlled trials. *BMJ* 2004; 329: 324–329.

21. Bandolier Extra. Topical analgesics: a review of reviews and a bit of perspective. March 2005. (www.jr2.ox.ac.uk/bandolier/Extrafrobando/Top extra3.pdf, accessed 24 Nov. 05)

22. Mason L, Moore RA, Edwards JE, *et al.* Systematic review of efficacy of topical rubefacients containing salicylates for the treatment of acute and chronic pain. *BMJ* 2004; 328: 998–1001.

23. Mason L, Moore RA, Derry S, *et al.* Systematic review of topical capsaicin for the treatment of chronic pain. *BMJ* 2004; 328: 991–995.

Pattern baldness

Pattern baldness (alopecia androgenetica) is a natural loss of hair associated with advancing age, usually developing in middle age, although the process can begin soon after puberty.

CAUSES

The precise biochemical mechanism is unknown, although it is believed to be a response to androgenic stimulation. The condition usually affects men, but women may also be affected.

TREATMENT – MINOXIDIL

Minoxidil 2% and 5% solutions are available without prescription for the treatment of pattern baldness.

Mode of action

Minoxidil is a potent, direct-acting peripheral vasodilator used in the treatment of hypertension. However, its use is limited by adverse effects, one of which is the encouragement of hair growth (hypertrichosis); it is this property that is exploited to treat baldness.

The mechanism of action is unknown, but regular application of minoxidil 2% solution causes some hair regrowth within 12 months. Clinical trials[1-4] have reported some hair regrowth in 20–90% of subjects, although a practising dermatologist reported that, in his experience, about 15% of patients experienced medium regrowth, while 50% experienced delayed hair loss and 35% continued to lose hair.[5] The manufacturer claims that the 5% solution can produce over 40% more hair growth over a 12-month period than the 2% solution, and that, in some cases, it produces visible hair growth at 8 weeks compared with 16 weeks for the regular strength solution.

Administration

For both strengths, 1 mL solution is applied to the affected area twice daily at 12-hourly intervals. The hair should not be washed for at least 1 hour after an application. The manufacturer claims that the solution is most likely to be effective in patients who have been losing their hair for fewer than 10 years and where the balding area is less than 10 cm diameter, and that it works in up to two-thirds of patients.

Reduction of hair loss is not visible for at least 4–6 weeks, and regrowth cannot be expected for at least 4 months with the 2% solution, but these periods may be reduced by as much as half with the 5% solution. New hair is soft and downy at first but will eventually become a normal thick growth in about one-third of the patients who respond to the treatment. Regrowth will only be maintained while the product is being used, and any regrown hair may be lost within 3–4 months of stopping treatment. The manufacturer recommends that treatment should be discontinued if there is no hair regrowth after 1 year. The product is relatively expensive and therefore requires financial commitment from the patient.

Contraindications, cautions and side-effects

The only contraindication to use is known sensitivity to minoxidil, or to ethanol or propylene glycol, which are included in the vehicle. Minoxidil is minimally absorbed through the scalp and topical application is unlikely to affect blood pressure, although patients with cardiovascular disease are advised to check with their doctor before using the product.

Use by pregnant or breastfeeding women is not advised, and the 5% solution should not be used at all by women. Side-effects in all body systems have been found to be equivalent to those of placebo, except for the skin, where more reactions such as local irritation, dryness and hair colour changes have been reported.

Products

- Regaine regular strength (2%)
- Regaine for Women (2%)
- Regaine Extra Strength (5%)
  All *Pfizer Consumer Healthcare*

PRODUCT SELECTION POINTS

Minoxidil 2% and 5% solutions are the only licensed products available. Some people may consider it worth paying up to around £300 a year indefinitely for its possible cosmetic benefits.

REFERENCES

1.   Savin RC. Use of topical minoxidil in the treatment of male pattern baldness. *J Am Acad Dermatol* 1987; 16: 696–704.
2.   Kuan YZ, Chen SY, Chen MJ, *et al.* Safety and efficacy of 2% topical minoxidil in the management of male pattern baldness in Chinese. *Changgeng Yi Xue Za Zhi* 1990; 13: 96–103.
3.   Connors TJ, Cooke DE, De Launey WE, *et al.* Australian trial of topical minoxidil and placebo in early male pattern baldness. *Australas J Dermatol* 1990; 31: 17–25.
4.   Karam P. Topical minoxidil therapy for androgenic alopecia in the Middle East. The Middle-Eastern Topical Minoxidil Study Group. *Int J Dermatol* 1993; 32: 763–766.
5.   Sinclair R. Male pattern androgenetic alopecia. *BMJ* 1998; 317: 865–869.

Premenstrual syndrome

Premenstrual syndrome (PMS) is associated with a wide range of physical and psychological symptoms, including fluid retention and oedema, breast tenderness, tension, anxiety and depression, all of which may appear up to 14 days before the start of a period and subside once menstruation commences. Symptoms vary between women and even from cycle to cycle.

CAUSES

The causes of PMS are still not known with certainty, but it is probably due to a range of metabolic factors influenced by hormones.

TREATMENT

Some over-the-counter treatments are available for PMS, for both specific and generalised symptoms. Ammonium chloride and caffeine are contained in a tablet marketed for water retention; pyridoxine is indicated for psychological and emotional symptoms, and evening primrose oil (EPO) for breast pain (cyclical mastalgia). However, in a condition with such broad symptoms and ill-defined causes, placebo effect is likely to play a large part in the perceived effectiveness of medication.

Ammonium chloride

Mode of action

Aqua Ban tablets (GR Lane) contain ammonium chloride, 325 mg, and caffeine, 100 mg, and the product is marketed as a mild diuretic for premenstrual water retention. Ammonium chloride is absorbed from the gastrointestinal tract and is converted into urea in the liver, which has the effect of acidifying the urine and producing transient diuresis. The caffeine content is equivalent to that in a cup of coffee; it has mild diuretic activity and is presumably also included as a stimulant to lift mood. Reducing sodium and water intake for a few days before a period may reduce fluid retention as effectively as over-the-counter medication.

Dosage, cautions and contraindications

The recommended dose is two tablets three times daily for 4 or 5 days before a period, stopping when menstruation starts. Ammonium chloride is irritant to the stomach, and to overcome this Aqua Ban tablets are enteric coated and it is recommended that they are taken after food. The product is contraindicated in patients with renal or hepatic impairment. Because it acidifies the urine, ammonium chloride may cause bladder inflammation, and excessive use may result in metabolic acidosis.

Pyridoxine (vitamin B6)

Mode of action

Pyridoxine is a co-enzyme in the final step of the biosynthesis of serotonin, a neurotransmitter known to have potent effects on mood. It has been postulated that a deficiency of pyridoxine may contribute to the depressive symptoms in PMS, and vitamin B6 has been found to relieve depression caused by oral contraceptives in some women. Clinical trials have produced conflicting evidence of effectiveness, but a meta-analysis[1] concluded that doses of vitamin B6 of up to 100 mg per day are likely to be of benefit in treating premenstrual symptoms and premenstrual depression.

There has been some controversy over the safety of pyridoxine. Pyridoxine is classified as General sale list (GSL), but high doses (2000–7000 mg daily) have been associated with peripheral neuropathies, which are generally reversible on discontinuation of the drug. In 1997, as a result over concerns about toxicity, the UK Government proposed the following restrictions on the availability and dosage of pyridoxine: preparations providing a daily dose of

50 mg and above to be classified as Prescription-only medicines, those providing 11–49 mg to be Pharmacy medicines; preparations containing up to 10 mg would be General sale list medicines. The Government was due to make a final decision in July 1998 but has not yet done so. The Royal Pharmaceutical Society has left pharmacists to decide for themselves whether to sell higher strengths of vitamin B6 as General sale list or Pharmacy medicines or to treat them as Prescription-only medicines. In the US, the daily maximum dose for preparations available without prescription has been set at 100 mg.

There are no longer any proprietary licensed medicines containing pyridoxine (apart from some multivitamin preparations containing very small amounts) but 10 mg, 20 mg and 50 mg non-proprietary tablets remain available. Proprietary products marketed as health supplements are also available.

Dosage

The recommended dose is 100–200 mg daily for 3 days before the onset of symptoms until 2 days after the start of menstruation, or 50–100 mg daily throughout the month. If no benefit is perceived within 3 months, treatment should be discontinued.

Evening primrose oil

Mode of action

EPO is a rich source of gamma-linolenic acid (GLA), a precursor of prostaglandin E_1, which is believed to be important in moderating responses to hormones associated with the menstrual cycle. One theory proposed to explain some of the symptoms of PMS is that sufferers have low levels of GLA. This deficiency is believed to be responsible for breast pain, as prostaglandin E is depleted and not available to down-regulate the response to prolactin, the hormone primarily responsible for lactation and which causes the breast engorgement and tenderness that some women experience before a period.

EPO was used to treat cyclical mastalgia and was licensed for this use and allowable on prescription. A systematic review[2] concluded that, on the limited evidence available, EPO was of little value in the management of PMS. All preparations of EPO have now been withdrawn and there are no licensed medicines containing it, although it remains available in products marketed as food supplements.

Agnus castus (chaste tree) fruit extract

The fruits of *Vitex agnus castus* (Verbenaceae) have traditionally been used to relieve the symptoms of PMS and other menstrual problems. Compounds similar in structure to the sex hormones have been isolated from some parts of the plant, and the effects of agnus castus have been described as similar to those of the corpus luteum. A prospective, randomised, placebo-controlled study published in 2001[3] found agnus castus to be considerably more effective than placebo across a wide range of premenstrual symptoms, at a dose standardised to 20 mg casticin (the active constituent) daily. Few adverse effects were reported. No preparations of agnus castus are available as licensed medicines, although products marketed as food supplements are available.

PRODUCT SELECTION POINTS

- There is some evidence of efficacy for vitamin B6 (pyridoxine) in premenstrual depression.
- Agnus castus fruit extract has traditionally been used in the treatment of PMS, and a placebo-controlled study found it to be effective against a wide range of symptoms.

PRODUCT RECOMMENDATIONS

- For premenstrual depression – vitamin B6 (pyridoxine) 100–200 mg daily on a cyclical basis for a few days around a period, or 50–100 mg daily continuously.
- For fluid retention and bloating – reduce sodium and fluid intake for a few days around a period; if this is unsuccessful and the problem is particularly troublesome, seek medical advice.
- For generalised symptoms – agnus castus is worth trying. It is only available as a food supplement, not as a licensed medicine.

REFERENCES

1. Wyatt KM, Dimmock PW, Jones PW, *et al*. Efficacy of vitamin B-6 in the treatment of premenstrual syndrome: systematic review. *BMJ* 1999; 318: 1375–1381.
2. Budeiri D, Li Wan Po A, Dornan JC. Is evening primrose oil of value in the treatment of premenstrual syndrome? *Control Clin Trials* 1996; 17: 60–68.
3. Schellenberg R. Treatment for the premenstrual syndrome with agnus castus fruit extract: prospective, randomised, placebo controlled study. *BMJ* 2001; 322: 134–137.

Scabies

Scabies is a contagious skin infestation caused by a mite.

The female scabies mite (*Sarcoptes scabei* var. hominis) burrows through the stratum corneum of the skin and lays its eggs just above the boundary between the epidermis and dermis. Sites of burrowing are mainly the finger webs and wrists, but can also be the palms of the hands, soles of the feet, external genitalia of both sexes and women's breasts. Mite burrows can sometimes be identified as slightly raised greyish 'pencil' lines, but they are not easy to spot. The principal symptom of infection is severe itching, caused by mite faeces or saliva containing water-soluble glycopeptides which eventually provoke an allergic response, although this takes several weeks to develop.

The areas of itching are not necessarily the same as the sites of infection but can be diffuse and widespread, and are often distributed symmetrically on both sides of the body. Symptoms are often as much a manifestation of damage done to the skin and secondary infection caused by scratching as of the infestation itself, and can be confused with excoriated eczema.

Skin contact for several minutes is necessary for transmission of infection from one person to another and often occurs through holding hands. Individuals may unwittingly spread infection for several weeks before symptoms develop, so treatment of all close contacts is necessary once infestation has been identified. The scabies mite cannot survive for long outside the human body and infection is not transferred through bedclothes or clothing.

Scabicidal preparations that are available without prescription contain one of the following:

- permethrin
- malathion
- benzyl benzoate
- crotamiton.

Antipruritic topical preparations, including those containing calamine and crotamiton, and systemic antihistamines can be used to treat the itching.

Relatively little clinical trial evidence for the efficacy of scabicides is available; some of the data that are available include drugs that are not licensed in the UK. There is evidence[1] that permethrin is more effective than crotamiton. Benzyl benzoate and permethrin have both been found to be effective, but permethrin produced less skin irritation and fewer eczematous reactions than benzyl benzoate.[2] Malathion and permethrin do not appear to have been directly compared for effectiveness, although case series reports with malathion[3] suggest that it is effective. The *British National Formulary* recommends permethrin as the first-choice treatment, and malathion if permethrin is inappropriate.

Permethrin

Mode of action, contraindications, cautions and side-effects

See chapter on Head lice.

Administration

The product is presented as a 5% cream. (The 1% cream rinse is licensed for head lice, and is not effective and should not be used for scabies.[4]) It is not licensed for use without prescription in children under 2 years of age, and treatment under medical supervision is advised for patients over 70 years and pregnant women.

Application is as for malathion (see below), but the preparation need only be left on the skin for 8–12 hours before being washed off.

For a single application of the cream, between 7.5 g for a 2-year-old child and 60 g for a large adult is required.

Product

There is only one product:

- Lyclear Dermal cream
  Chefaro UK

Malathion

Mode of action, contraindications, cautions and side-effects

See chapter on Head lice.

Administration

The lotion preparations licensed for the treatment of scabies are the same as those for head lice, but the method of administration is different. Products are licensed for use without prescription from the age of 6 months. They may also be used in pregnancy, but treatment under medical supervision is advisable. Use of the alcohol-based lotion on skin damaged by scratching should be avoided, as it can cause stinging.

The lotion should be applied with the hand, cotton wool, a small sponge or an 8 cm paintbrush to cool, dry and clean skin. Traditional advice to have a hot bath before application has now been discounted, as this does not increase the effectiveness of the scabicide, and may in fact decrease it by enhancing absorption into the blood stream and away from the site of action on the skin. The lotion should be applied to the entire body surface from the soles of the feet to the hairline, including the groin, axillae and skin folds, between fingers and toes, and under finger and toe nails. Lotion should be re-applied to the hands if they are washed after application.

Traditional advice that the head and neck do not need to be treated is incorrect, as mites can be present on the face and ears, particularly in the elderly and young children; missing out these areas can therefore lead to treatment failure. About 100 mL malathion lotion is needed for a single application for an average adult. Mites are usually killed within minutes, but the aqueous lotion should be left on for 24 hours and the alcoholic lotion for 12 hours, to ensure complete eradication. Two applications, a week apart, are now recommended for both permethrin and malathion. Itching may persist for up to 2–3 weeks until the allergenic mite material is cleared from the skin, and should not be regarded as a sign of treatment failure. Patients should therefore be reassured and symptomatic relief offered, if necessary.

Treatment failure may have occurred if itching has not ceased after 3 weeks, or if new areas of itching continue to appear 7–10 days after treatment. In these situations, patients should be referred to their doctor for confirmation of the diagnosis, in which case a second application of scabicide may be advised. If treatment fails for a second time, patients should be referred to a dermatologist.

Products

- Aqueous solutions (0.5%)
    — Derbac-M liquid
      SSL International
    — Quellada M liquid
      GSK Consumer Healthcare

- Alcoholic solution (0.5%)
    — Prioderm lotion
      SSL International

Benzyl benzoate

Benzyl Benzoate Application BP, a 25% emulsion, was at one time the first-choice treatment for scabies, but it can be unpleasant to use and has now been superseded by more effective products. At least two, and sometimes three, consecutive applications of benzyl benzoate, left on for 24 hours each, may be necessary to eradicate mite infestations. In addition, benzyl benzoate has an unpleasant smell, is irritant, can cause itching, burning and stinging, and may cause skin rashes. It should not be used on patients with skin excoriated through scratching.

For children, it has been suggested that the emulsion can be diluted to reduce adverse effects, but this also reduces efficacy. The *British National Formulary* recommends that benzyl benzoate should not be used at all for children.

Products

- Benzyl Benzoate Application BP
- Ascabiol emulsion
  Sanofi-Aventis

Crotamiton

Crotamiton has antipruritic and weak scabicidal activity. However, up to five 24-hour applications at daily intervals are necessary for complete eradication of infections. Crotamiton is recommended for controlling residual itching after treatment with a more effective scabicide. It appears to have a relatively long duration of activity of 6–10 hours, requiring application only two or three times a day. One trial[5] found it to be less effective in reducing pruritus than permethrin.

Product

There is only one product:

- Eurax cream and lotion (10%)
  Novartis Consumer Health

PRODUCT SELECTION POINTS

- Malathion and permethrin both appear to be effective as scabicides, and are the treatments of choice. There is no firm evidence that one is more effective than the other.
- Permethrin cream is 3–4 times more expensive per treatment than malathion preparations.
- Unlike the case with head lice, all close contacts of a person infected with scabies should be treated.
- Residual itch following treatment is not necessarily a sign of treatment failure. Symptomatic treatment can be recommended for itching; systemic antihistamines are probably most effective, although topical application of calamine lotion or crotamiton cream or lotion may also be helpful.

PRODUCT RECOMMENDATIONS

- First choice for eradication of infection –permethrin cream or malathion preparations.
- For treatment of residual pruritus – a systemic antihistamine, with additional application of calamine lotion or crotamiton cream or lotion, if desired.

REFERENCES

1. Walker GJA, Johnstone PW. Interventions for treating scabies. *The Cochrane Library*, issue 3. Chichester, UK: John Wiley & Sons, 2003 (www.thecochranelibrary.com).
2. Haustein UF, Hlawa B. Treatment of scabies with permethrin versus lindane and benzyl benzoate. *Acta Derm Venereol* 1989; 69: 348–351.
3. Walker G, Johnstone P. Scabies. *Clin Evid* 2002: 1543–1548. (www.clinical evidence.com/ceweb/conditions/skd/1707/1707_I4.jsp, accessed 28 Nov. 05)
4. Cox NH. Permethrin treatment in scabies infestation: importance of the correct formulation. *BMJ* 2000; 320: 37–8.
5. Taplin D, Meinking TL, Chen JA, Sanchez R. Comparison of crotamiton 10% cream (Eurax) and permethrin 5% cream (Elimite) for the treatment of scabies in children. *Pediatr Dermatol* 1990; 7: 67–73.

Smoking cessation products

Smoking of cigarettes, and to a lesser extent cigar and pipe smoking, are not in themselves diseases but the consequences of smoking, in terms of mortality, suffering and financial costs, are comparable to any pandemic. Persuading and helping smokers to give up is one of the greatest challenges facing healthcare professionals – one that pharmacists are ideally place to meet, with their ready accessibility to the public and a range of effective smoking cessation aids available without prescription.

ADVERSE EFFECTS OF TOBACCO SMOKE

The constituents of tobacco smoke include nicotine and about 4000 pyrolysis products, including tar components (aliphatic and aromatic hydrocarbons, phenols and other compounds), alcohols, amines, nitrosamines, ammonia, nitrogen oxides and carbon monoxide.

Nicotine

Nicotine is the addictive component of tobacco smoke. It is readily absorbed through the oral mucosa and the lungs, and peak blood concentrations are achieved very rapidly – within 30 seconds of a puff of a cigarette. The drug acts on the central nervous system, causing transient euphoria, a feeling of relaxation, improved concentration and memory, and reduced appetite. Nicotine is highly addictive, producing withdrawal symptoms of anxiety, difficulty in concentrating and irritability, which are relieved by the next cigarette. Eventually smokers establish a steady blood concentration of nicotine through a regular smoking pattern, preventing withdrawal cravings.

Psychological and behavioural components contribute to dependence on smoking in approximately equal measure to physiological addiction, and are of two types: associations that reinforce the habit, which can be positive (e.g. social drinking and following meals) or negative (e.g. stressful situations), and ritual behaviour associated with lighting, holding and inhaling a cigarette, which the smoker associates with the reward of a measure of nicotine.

Other effects of nicotine include stimulation of the autonomic nervous system, which increases heart rate, raises blood pressure and causes vasoconstriction. It also increases the stickiness of blood platelets, leading to increased risk of clotting. Nicotine raises the levels of serotonin, catecholamines, pituitary hormones and vaso-pressin in the blood and brain. It also increases gastric acid secretion, which may lead to peptic ulceration.

Tar

Tobacco tar is a complex mixture of compounds, many of which are carcinogenic. Tar is largely unabsorbed and most becomes trapped in the lungs, causing carcinomas; the increased risk of bronchial carci-nomas compared with non-smokers ranges from 15-fold for someone who regularly smokes fewer than ten cigarettes a day to 60-fold for someone who smokes more than 40 cigarettes a day. The risk of cancer of the buccal cavity, larynx and oesophagus is also much higher than for the population as a whole. Some tar constituents enter the blood stream and pass through the kidneys, bladder and liver and can be responsible for cancer in these organs.

Carbon monoxide

Carbon monoxide binds tightly to haemoglobin, forming carboxy-haemoglobin and decreasing the availability of oxygen in the blood supply to the tissues, including the myocardium. Carbon monoxide acts together with nicotine to significantly increase the risk of ischaemic heart disease. Circulatory problems can also lead to inter-mittent claudication, which can lead to gangrene and result in limb amputation.

Other effects

Tobacco smoke irritates the upper airways and inhibits the protective actions of the ciliary epithelium and the production of mucus by glandular cells. This leads to chronic pharyngitis, laryngitis and, in particular, bronchitis. Eventual destruction of bronchial and alveolar tissues often results, leading to bronchiectasis and emphysema, irreversible conditions that progressively restrict gaseous interchange in the lungs and cause increasing respiratory distress.

Smoking can also damage the retina and optic nerve, increase blood sugar and lipid levels, have teratogenic effects in both men and women, increasing the possibility of congenital malformations in babies, increase the likelihood of premature birth and decrease birth weight.

TREATMENT – NICOTINE REPLACEMENT THERAPY

Giving up smoking is essentially a matter of self-motivation and determination and most ex-smokers have stopped without using drugs or any kind of assistance. Nevertheless, use of nicotine-replacement products (NRT) products, which partially replace nicotine from smoking in a regimen that gradually reduces nicotine intake to zero, have been shown to be helpful and are available for those who feel unable to give up unaided. Presentations include chewing gum, transdermal patches, a cigarette-shaped inhaler, a sublingual tablet, a lozenge and a nasal spray.

There is strong evidence that all forms of NRT are effective as part of a strategy to promote smoking cessation; they increase the odds of quitting by 1.5–2-fold, regardless of setting.[1] Furthermore, the effectiveness of NRT appears to be largely independent of the intensity of additional support provided to the smoker.[2-5]

Mode of action

NRT assists smokers to give up by providing nicotine, although at a lower level than is obtained through smoking, to help prevent withdrawal symptoms and cravings. After a period at a steady state, nicotine intake is progressively reduced to zero over 2–3 months. Nicotine is absorbed efficiently through the buccal and nasal mucosae, the skin and the lungs, all of which are utilised for NRT products.

Delivery systems

Transdermal patches

There are two types of transdermal patch, both of which are changed daily: one is left on for 24 hours; the other is used for 16 hours daily during waking hours only and is removed before going to bed. The former provides a residual nicotine level the next morning and may be better for smokers who crave a cigarette as soon as they wake up. However, nicotine levels maintained overnight can produce sleep disturbances and should be avoided by use of the 16-hour patch. Three brands of patch are available, all available in three strengths, which are intended to allow for a smooth reduction in nicotine intake (see below). With both 16- and 24-hour patches, nicotine plasma concentrations are about half of those obtained from smoking the average number of cigarettes per day.

Chewing gum

Nicotine is absorbed from chewing gum through the buccal mucosa; peak blood concentrations are reached within about 2 minutes and the contents of a piece of gum are intended to be released over about 30 minutes. A piece of gum is chewed whenever the urge to smoke is felt, and the method mimics the pattern of nicotine intake obtained by smoking, but peak blood level are lower and the steady-state nicotine concentration is about 30% of that obtained from cigarettes. The method is also useful because putting a piece of gum in the mouth and chewing provides some of the same kind of behavioural involvement as smoking.

Inhaler

The inhaler is intended to address both the physical and behavioural components of smoking cessation, as it involves putting the inhaler to the mouth and inhaling as in smoking; it may be particularly useful for the highly behaviour-dependent smoker. Nicotine is contained in an impregnated porous polyethylene plug inside a plastic tube, and is used in the same way as a cigarette, with 'puffs' being inhaled as desired. Users can inhale by deep pulmonary inhalation or shallow buccal 'puffing'. Nicotine intake is slightly higher with the former method, but both types produce comparable steady-state plasma concentrations equivalent to those achieved with nicotine gum.

Sublingual tablets

This presentation provides an unobtrusive method of nicotine replacement. One sublingual tablet is bioequivalent to one piece of nicotine 2 mg chewing gum, and the recommended dosage is comparable. Like lozenges (see below), it may be a useful method for smokers who do not like or have difficulty in chewing gum.

Nasal spray

This presentation was developed to provide a fast-acting and flexible method of nicotine delivery for highly dependent smokers. A 50-microlitre metered spray, administered to each nostril, delivers a nicotine dose of 1 mg. Nicotine is rapidly absorbed from the nasal mucosa, reaching maximum plasma levels in 10–15 minutes; about half the dose is absorbed. Side-effects include nose and throat irritation, watering eyes and coughing, and are fairly common, especially in the first couple of weeks of treatment.

Lozenges

As with chewing gum, nicotine is absorbed from lozenges through the buccal mucosa and these are used in much the same way. Lozenges provide a more discreet means of NRT than chewing gum, and may be preferred by those who do not like or have difficulty chewing gum. Two brands are available.

- Nicotinell Mint 1 mg lozenges (Novartis Consumer Health) contain 1 mg nicotine and are more or less bioequivalent to 2 mg gum, as some nicotine remains bound to the ion-exchange resin in the latter and is not released.
- NiQuitin CQ Lozenges (GSK Consumer Healthcare) are available in 2 mg and 4 mg strengths.

Relative effectiveness of presentations

The odds ratios (ORs) of effectiveness of NRT presentations[1] are given in the table below.

Relative effectiveness of NRT presentations

Presentation	OR (95% CI)
Patches	1.81 (1.63, 2.02)
*Gum	1.66 (1.52, 1.81)
Nasal spray	2.14 (1.44, 3.18)
Sublingual tablet/lozenge	2.05 (1.62, 2.59)

OR is the ratio of smokers who, in clinical trials, have stopped smoking as a result of using a particular NRT presentation against those who have given up without using anything. 95% confidence intervals [95% CI] give the limits within which the true value of the OR will be expected to be included in 95% of cases.
*In highly dependent smokers there was a significant benefit of 4 mg gum compared with 2 mg gum (OR 2.20, 95% CI: 1.85, 3.25).

Dosage and administration

Subjects should stop smoking completely while using any NRT product, and different presentations should not be used together. (In 2005 a licensing variation was obtained for Nicorette gum and inhalator permitting use for smoking reduction before a quit attempt – see below.)

Transdermal patches

Transdermal patches have the convenience of a once-daily application and may be the most suitable form of NRT for people in whom the behavioural aspects of smoking is relatively unimportant. All three of the available brands (Nicorette [Pfizer Consumer Healthcare], Nicotinell TTS [Novartis Consumer Health] and NiQuitin CQ [GSK Consumer Healthcare]) are supplied in three strengths. The three strengths of Nicotinell TTS and NiQuitin CQ provide 7, 14 and 21 mg nicotine over 24 hours. Nicorette patches deliver 5, 10 and 15 mg over the 16 hours daily for which they are intended to be applied, and overnight plasma nicotine levels should be insignificant.

The recommended starting strength for all the brands is generally the highest, except for light smokers (defined as fewer than ten cigarettes per day for NiQuitin CQ, and fewer than 20 per day for Nicotinell TTS), for whom the medium strength should be used first. The recommended treatment period and the length of time on each strength varies between brands, but the overall strategy is a stabilisation period on the high strength for 4–8 weeks, followed by a progressive stepping down of strength over a further 2–8 weeks, before stopping altogether. The total maximum recommended course is 12 weeks for Nicorette and Nicotinell TTS and 10 weeks for NiQuitin CQ.

Transdermal patches should be applied daily to a clean, dry, non-hairy area of the trunk or upper arm. Nicorette patches should be removed at bedtime and a fresh one applied next morning. To minimise the possibility of localised skin reaction, a new site of application should be chosen each day, and several days should be allowed to elapse before a patch is re-applied to the same area. Used patches should be folded in half with the adhesive side inwards and disposed of carefully, because they still contain significant amounts of nicotine, certainly sufficient to poison a child.

Chewing gum

Use of nicotine chewing gum mimics the pattern of peaks and troughs of nicotine provided by smoking, although blood levels achieved are much lower. Because a piece of gum can be chewed whenever the urge to smoke is felt, the method may be most suitable for the smoker who finds cigarette cravings difficult to resist. It may also provide a greater sense of control over curbing the habit, and the chewing activity also acts as a behavioural substitute for smoking.

Nicotine gum is available in two brands (Nicorette [Pfizer Consumer Healthcare] and Nicotinell [Novartis Consumer Health]), both in two strengths: 2 mg and 4 mg. Recommended dosages and maxima differ slightly for the two brands.

- **For Nicorette,** heavier smokers (more than 20 cigarettes per day) and those who crave a cigarette within 20 minutes of waking up should start on the higher strength. Less heavy smokers should start with the lower strength, and transfer to the higher if they need more than 15 pieces per day. A piece may be chewed whenever the urge to smoke is felt. The recommended daily maximum is 15 pieces per day for both strengths.
- **For Nicotinell,** for both strengths, one piece of gum is to be chewed when the urge to smoke is felt. The normal requirement is 8–12 pieces daily, but a maximum of 25 × 2 mg or 15 × 4 mg pieces daily may be used. The higher strength is recommended if particularly strong withdrawal symptoms are experienced.

For both brands, the recommended course of chewing gum is about 3 months' *ad libitum* use, after which it is gradually withdrawn over a few weeks. For smoking reduction before attempting to give up, Nicorette gum may be used between smoking episodes. A quit attempt should be made as soon as the smoker feels ready. Professional advice should be sought if there has been no reduction in smoking after 6 weeks or no quit attempt within 9 months.

Correct chewing technique maximises buccal absorption of nicotine from the gum and reduces adverse effects from swallowing the drug in saliva. The gum is chewed slowly to release nicotine, until the taste becomes strong and 'peppery'. Chewing is then stopped and the gum is rested between the gum and cheek until the taste fades. This procedure is repeated until the gum has lost its flavour, which should take about 30 minutes.

Inhaler

Because the device (Nicorette Inhalator [Pfizer Consumer Healthcare]) is held like a cigarette and the nicotine is inhaled by puffing, the nicotine inhaler provides a close approximation of the hand-to-mouth activity and inhaling associated with smoking that reinforce the nicotine addiction. This presentation is therefore recommended for highly behavioural-dependent smokers. *Ad libitum* usage also helps to alleviate cravings and provides a sense of control. Nicorette Inhalator may be used in the same way as Nicorette gum for smoking reduction before a quit attempt (see above).

The device consists of a two-part plastic mouthpiece and holder, into which is inserted a cartridge containing a polyethylene porous plug impregnated with nicotine. Each plug contains 10 mg, 5 mg of which is available for inhalation. Each puff delivers about 13 micrograms nicotine, which is only 4–8% of that obtained per puff of a cigarette. However, a plug will last much longer than a cigarette because the available nicotine content is designed to be released over about 20 minutes of active continuous puffing but, as in smoking, puffs are only taken intermittently. In this way, nicotine intake is not only reduced compared with cigarettes, but the concentration peaks are flattened. The plug is flavoured with menthol, and the disappearance of the flavour indicates that the nicotine is exhausted.

Usage is 6–12 cartridges per day. The inhaler is intended to be used freely for 3 months, following which the daily dosage should be reduced over a further 6–8 weeks. Treatment should be completed within 6 months.

Sublingual tablets

A sublingual tablet (Nicorette Microtab [Pfizer Consumer Healthcare]) is placed under the tongue, where it slowly disintegrates in about 30 minutes. One tablet is used per hour (8–12 tablets per day), or two per hour (16–24 tablets per day) for heavy smokers (more than 20 cigarettes per day). The dose may be increased to two per hour if one seems inadequate to control craving, or if the individual feels that relapse is likely. The absolute maximum dosage is 40 tablets per day. The full dosage should be maintained for 3 months, and then gradually tapered off to zero within the next 3 months.

Nasal spray

One metered spray (Nicorette Nasal Spray [Pfizer Consumer Health-care]) is inhaled into each nostril when necessary to relieve craving, with a maximum rate of two doses per hour and 64 sprays (32 into each nostril) in 24 hours. *Ad libitum* dosage can be maintained for up to 8 weeks, after which the dosage should be reduced by half over the next 2 weeks, and down to zero over the following 2 weeks.

Lozenges

Products include:

- Nicotinell Mint (1 mg lozenge)
  Novartis Consumer Health

- NiQuitin CQ (2 mg and 4 mg lozenge)
  GSK Consumer Healthcare.

The dosage schedule for Nicotinell lozenges is much the same as for Nicotinell gum: one lozenge every 1–2 hours, when the urge to smoke is felt. The recommended daily dosage is 8–12 lozenges, but a maximum of 25 may be used. The sucking technique is similar to that for nicotine chewing gum: a lozenge is sucked slowly until the taste becomes strong; it is then 'parked' between the cheek and gum until the taste has faded, and the procedure continued until the lozenge has gone. One lozenge should last for about half an hour.

For NiQuitin CQ Lozenges the strength required is determined by the time between waking and the first cigarette, rather than by the number of cigarettes smoked per day as for other NRT products. The 4 mg lozenge is recommended for those who smoke within 30 minutes of waking, and the 2 mg strength for those who are less dependent and can wait longer before smoking their first cigarette of the day. Users stay on the same strength of lozenge throughout the course, stepping down the frequency of use rather than the strength of the preparation. The total length of treatment is up to 24 weeks, starting with one lozenge every 1–2 hours, to a maximum of 15 lozenges per day, for the first 6 weeks, reducing to one lozenge every 2–4 hours for the next two 3-week periods, then to one every 4–8 hours. There-after, one or two lozenges may be sucked when the urge to smoke is strong, and use should have ceased altogether within a further 12 weeks.

Cautions, contraindications and adverse effects

NRT products provide much lower doses of nicotine than are obtained by smoking, and the adverse effects are not complicated by the additional toxic effects of tar and carbon monoxide generated in tobacco smoke. Nevertheless, because of the cardiovascular effects of nicotine, caution is advised with the use of NRT products in patients with a history of angina, recent myocardial infarction or cerebrovas-cular accident, cardiac arrhythmias, hypertension or peripheral vas-cular disease. Because of the effects of nicotine on metabolism, caution is also advised in patients with diabetes, hyperthyroidism or phaeochromocytoma.

With the use of patches, there is a possibility of localised skin reactions, and they should be avoided by patients with any chronic or serious skin condition.

Although nicotine can exacerbate symptoms in patients with peptic ulcers or gastritis, the possibility is greater with gum than other NRT products, as nicotine may be swallowed and enter the stomach directly. Denture wearers may also have difficulty in chewing gum.

Patients with chronic bronchitis or severe asthma may find inhalation from the inhaler difficult, and should therefore avoid this product.

In addition to the potential adverse effects mentioned, NRT products may produce the same range of side-effects as nicotine from smoking and these include hiccups, sore throat, headache, nausea and dizziness. However, these are less likely to occur than with smoking, and clinical trials have shown most to be comparable to those caused by placebo. Nicotine withdrawal symptoms such as somnolence, impaired concentration, mood swings, fatigue, hunger, productive cough, bowel disturbances and paraesthesia are also possible.

From January 2006, following advice from a working group of the Committee on Safety of Medicines on NRT, supply without prescription was extended to 'risk' groups to which supply was previously permitted only on the authorisation of a doctor. These groups are: pregnant and breastfeeding women, adolescents aged 12–18 years, and smokers with underlying disease such as cardiovascular, hepatic and renal disease, diabetes mellitus and those taking concurrent medication.

Transfer of dependence from smoking to NRT products is unlikely, but possible.

Interactions

The only interaction that is possibly directly attributable to NRT is with adenosine, although this appears only to have occurred experimentally in healthy subjects, when concurrent use of nicotine gum, 2 mg, with adenosine raised blood pressure, increased heart rate and produced angina-like chest pain.

Tobacco smoke reduces serum levels of a wide range of drugs and adjustment of dosage may be necessary when smokers have given up. The *British National Formulary* specifically cites theophylline, but dose adjustment may also be required for beta-blockers, adrenergic agonists, nifedipine, tricyclic antidepressants, phenothiazines, benzodiazepines and insulin.

TREATMENT – NICOBREVIN

Nicobrevin (Cedar Health) is a 28-day course of gelatin capsules containing menthyl valerate, quinine, camphor and eucalyptus oil. The rationale given by the original manufacturer for the formulation was that quinine helps to alleviate the effects of smoking withdrawal on tobacco craving and metabolism; camphor helps to alleviate the undesirable effects of smoking on the respiratory system; menthyl valerate is a mild sedative and helps to relieve the irritability experienced by persons giving up smoking; oil of eucalyptus helps to relieve the accumulation of mucus that occurs during smoking withdrawal. These claimed actions remain to be substantiated, but the complex dosage regimen is likely to enhance the product's attention-placebo effect. One small-scale, placebo-controlled, double-blind trial[6] of Nicobrevin reported that it was significantly superior to placebo as an aid to smoking cessation, and that the product was rated by subjects as 'very effective'.

PRODUCT SELECTION POINTS

- Motivation is the most important factor in giving up smoking, but NRT has been clinically proven to be an effective aid.
- Low-dependency smokers who are highly motivated to give up probably do not need any kind of smoking-cessation aid.
- Lozenges provide the lowest dose of nicotine of all NRT products and may be useful for light smokers who feel they need some pharmacological as well as psychological support.
- There is little difference in efficacy overall between the various forms of NRT, but a particular form or strength may be best suited to a particular type of smoker.
- Patches are convenient to use, but may not be suitable for smokers with a high behavioural component to their dependence.
- The 24-hour patch is better for smokers who crave a cigarette within 20 minutes of waking up in the morning, otherwise the 16-hour and 24-hour patches are equally suitable and effective. The 16-hour patch should be used if sleep disturbances occur with the 24-hour patch.
- Gum of 4 mg strength is probably the best approach for heavy smokers with high behavioural dependence; the 2 mg strength is suitable for moderate and relatively light smokers.
- The nicotine inhaler might be most useful for moderate smokers with high behavioural dependency.
- The nasal spray may be the most effective form of NRT for very heavily dependent smokers.

- There is insufficient trial evidence to confirm the effectiveness of Nicobrevin.

PRODUCT RECOMMENDATIONS

NRT is the smoking-cessation treatment of choice. The following recommendations are made for specific types of smoker:

- Low dependency (fewer than ten cigarettes per day); high motivation – encouragement and advice only.
- Low dependency – lozenges, sublingual tablets or 2 mg gum.
- Moderate dependency (10–20 cigarettes per day), with low behavioural component and normal or heavy build – patch, starting with highest strength.
- Moderate dependency, low behavioural component, slight build – patch, starting with middle strength.
- Moderate dependency, high behavioural component – inhaler, sublingual tablets or 2 mg gum (switch to 4 mg if necessary).
- High dependency (more than 20 cigarettes per day) – 4 mg gum or lozenges or nasal spray.
- Very high dependency – nasal spray.

REFERENCES

1. Silagy C, Lancaster T, Stead L, *et al.* Nicotine replacement therapy for smoking cessation. *The Cochrane Library,* issue 3. Chichester, UK: John Wiley & Sons, 2004 (www.thecochranelibrary.com).
2. Lancaster T, Stead LF. Physician advice for smoking cessation. *The Cochrane Library,* issue 4. Chichester, UK: John Wiley & Sons, 2004 (www.thecochranelibrary.com).
3. Sinclair HK, Bond CM, Stead LF. Community pharmacy personnel interventions for smoking cessation. *The Cochrane Library,* issue 1. Chichester, UK: John Wiley & Sons, 2006 (www.thecochranelibrary.com).
4. Lancaster T, Stead LF. Individual behavioural counselling for smoking cessation. In: *The Cochrane Library,* issue 3. Chichester, UK: John Wiley & Sons, 2004 (www.thecochranelibrary.com).

5.   Rice VH, Stead LF. Nursing interventions for smoking cessation. *The Cochrane Library*, issue 3. Chichester, UK: John Wiley & Sons, 2004 (www.thecochranelibrary.com).

6.   Dankwa E, Perry L, Perkins A. A double-blind, placebo-controlled study to determine the efficacy of Nicobrevin anti-smoking capsules. *Br J Clin Pract* 1988; 42: 359–363.

Sore throat

Sore throat as a symptom of the common cold is treated using one or more of the following approaches: stimulation of saliva production, use of antimicrobials and local anaesthesia. Although many products for sore throat contain antibacterial compounds, causative organisms are usually viruses and are therefore not susceptible to these. A systematic review of randomised controlled trials[1] concluded that systemic aspirin, ibuprofen and paracetamol are at least as effective as products marketed specifically for sore throat.

TREATMENT – PASTILLES AND LOZENGES

The action of sucking anything produces saliva, which lubricates and soothes inflamed tissues and washes infecting organisms off them. All lozenges and pastilles, regardless of ingredients, produce this action and much, if not all, of their effectiveness is due to this.

Demulcents

Non-medicated glycogelatin-based demulcent pastilles, such as Glycerin, Lemon and Honey Pastilles or boiled sweets, may be as effective as anything for soothing a sore throat, for the reasons stated above. Because they contain no medicament, they can be taken as often as necessary to stop the throat feeling dry, thereby relieving discomfort. Some products contain ingredients with volatile constituents, particularly eucalyptus oil and menthol. These produce a sensation of clearing blocked nasal and upper respiratory passages, and can be useful in relieving symptoms of upper respiratory tract infections that often accompany sore throat. The main disadvantage of demulcent throat lozenges and pastilles is their high sugar content.

Product examples

- Glycerin, Lemon and Honey Pastilles

- Meggezones Pastilles
  Schering-Plough

- Potter's Sore Throat Pastilles
  Ernest Jackson

- Zubes
  Ernest Jackson

Antibacterials

The compounds used in sore throat lozenges are mainly cationic surfactants and phenolic antiseptics. They are bactericidal and have varying degrees of antifungal activity. They possess activity against lipophilic viruses; however, the rhinoviruses that are largely responsible for the common cold are hydrophilic. A sore throat complicated by a secondary bacterial infection would normally be treated with a systemic antibiotic. Several sugar-free antibacterial throat lozenges are available.

Product examples

- Benzalkonium chloride
  - Bradosol Sugar-free Lozenges
    Novartis Consumer Health

- Dequalinium chloride
  - Dequadin
    Crookes

- Cetylpyridinium chloride
  - Merocets
    SSL International

- Amylmetacresol
  - Strepsils
    Crookes

- Hexylresorcinol
  - Lemsip Sore Throat Antibacterial Lozenges Honey and Lemon
    Reckitt Benckiser
  - TCP Sore Throat Lozenges
    Chefaro

- Tyrothricin
  - Tyrozets
    McNeil

Local anaesthetics

Benzocaine is now the only local anaesthetic used in throat lozenges and is included in several products that may prove useful if the patient finds swallowing uncomfortable. Concentrations vary between 5 and 10 mg per lozenge, which is within the therapeutic dose range. Local anaesthetics are effective when applied to the oral mucosa, and may provide additional relief for patients with more seriously inflamed throats that make swallowing painful. Local anaesthetics can cause sensitisation in some individuals with prolonged use, so usage should be limited to 5 days. They should not be used at all by children or the elderly.

Product examples

The following contain benzocaine.

- Dequacaine
  Crookes

- Merocaine
  SSL International

- Tyrozets
  McNeil

Product

- Strefen
  Crookes

Flurbiprofen

Flurbiprofen is a non-steroidal anti-inflammatory drug (NSAID) that is available as a lozenge formulation for the relief of sore throat. In a double-blind trial,[2] flurbiprofen lozenges were found to be effective and well tolerated. The dosage is one lozenge every 3–6 hours to a maximum of five lozenges in 24 hours. The usual precautions for the use of NSAIDs apply.

TREATMENT – GARGLES

Gargles mainly contain antiseptic ingredients, often the same as those in throat lozenges, with the same drawback insofar as most have no proven antiviral activity. In addition, contact time with infected tissue is extremely short. The main action of gargles is the mechanical removal of microbes from the pharynx, but tests have shown that levels of contamination are restored within about an hour.

Product examples

- Oraldene (contains hexetidine)
  Pfizer Consumer Healthcare

- TCP liquid antiseptic (contains phenol and halogenated phenols)
  Chefaro UK

- Difflam sore throat rinse (contains benzydamine, an
  anti-inflammatory)
  3M

- Betadine gargle and mouthwash (contains 1% povidone-iodine; the
  iodine content renders it unsuitable for patients with thyroid problems or
  those on lithium therapy, and in pregnant and breastfeeding women)
  Medlock

TREATMENT – SPRAYS

AAA Mouth and Throat Spray (Manx) and Ultra Chloraseptic Anaesthetic Spray (Prestige Brands) both contain benzocaine (3 mg per recommended adult dose) and may be used for children aged 6 years and over. Eludril Spray (Ceuta) contains chlorhexidine and tetracaine; it is recommended for adult use only.

PRODUCT SELECTION POINTS

- The greatest beneficial effect of most throat lozenges may result from the salivation produced by sucking them; the active ingredients are less important.
- Antiseptic constituents of throat lozenges probably have little impact on the causative organisms of sore throat.
- Gargles may have little effect beyond transient relief.
- Anaesthetic constituents of lozenges and sprays relieve discomfort but can cause sensitisation.

PRODUCT RECOMMENDATIONS

- For a sore, 'tickly' throat – demulcent pastilles (e.g. Glycerin, Lemon and Honey).
- For a sore throat with discomfort on swallowing – lozenges containing benzocaine or flurbiprofen.

REFERENCES

1. Thomas M, Del Mar C, Glasziou P. How effective are treatments other than antibiotics for acute sore throat? *Br J Gen Pract* 2000; 50: 817–820.
2. Watson N, Nimmo WS, Christian J, *et al*. Relief of sore throat with the anti-inflammatory throat lozenge flurbiprofen 8.75 mg: a randomised, double-blind, placebo-controlled study of efficacy and safety. *Int J Clin Pract* 2000; 54: 490–496.

Temporary sleep disturbance

Temporary sleep disturbance (insomnia) is reported by nearly one-third of adults and there is a high demand for hypnotics. Expansion of the market for non-prescription hypnotics, with the launch of several new antihistamine brands, appeared to coincide with the reduction in prescribed hypnotics, following discouragement by medical authorities of prescribing benzodiazepines in particular, after it became apparent that widespread and long-term use was leading to problems of tolerance and dependence. Although non-prescription sleep aids are quite safe when used for limited periods according to manufacturers' directions, there is still the danger of developing tolerance and psychological dependence if they are relied on as a long-term solution to an insomnia problem that may have underlying organic or psychological causes.

Over-the-counter hypnotics should only be recommended when the normal sleep pattern has been disturbed for an identifiable reason (e.g. long-haul air travel, a change in shift-working patterns or a stressful situation of short duration).

TREATMENT – ANTIHISTAMINES

Compounds available

Compounds available are:

- diphenhydramine hydrochloride
- promethazine hydrochloride.

Mode of action

The relevant actions of antihistamines are described in the chapter on Cough. The effectiveness of antihistamines as hypnotics may relate to their antimuscarinic actions, but it has also been proposed that sedation is caused by blockade of central H_1-receptors.

Diphenhydramine hydrochloride

Diphenhydramine is a potent antihistamine of the ethanolamine group, with a high incidence of sedation and antimuscarinic effects. Maximum sedation is achieved 1–4 hours after administration, and duration of sedation is 3–6 hours. From psychomotor tests it appears that mental alertness and cognitive ability are not impaired beyond the length of time that drowsiness lasts. The optimum dose appears to be 50 mg; higher doses do not increase efficacy but do increase the potential for side-effects.

Dosage

Adults over 16 years – 50 mg at bedtime.

Products

- Dreemon tablets (25 mg) and syrup (10 mg per 5 mL)
  Peach Pharmaceuticals

- Nytol tablets (25 mg)
- Nytol One-A-Night tablets (50 mg)
  both *GSK Consumer Healthcare*

- Paxidorm tablets (25 mg)
  Norma Chemicals

- Panadol Night Pain tablets (diphenhydramine 25 mg and paracetamol 500 mg)
  GSK Consumer Healthcare

Promethazine hydrochloride

Promethazine hydrochloride is a phenothiazine derivative with marked sedative properties. It is long acting, with action reported to last 4–12 hours. Residual drowsiness the next morning therefore seems more likely than with diphenhydramine.

Dosage

Adults over 16 years – 20 or 25 mg, depending on brand, at bedtime.

Promethazine Oral Solution BP (Phenergan Elixir) is licensed as a Pharmacy medicine with a sedative dosage for children as follows: 2–5 years of age, 15–20 mg; 5–10 years of age, 20–25 mg, as a single night-time dose. The preparation can only be given to children between 1 and 2 years of age under medical supervision. It is not recommended for children under 12 months, as it is thought that giving any sedative drug, including phenothiazines, to an infant may increase the risk of sudden infant death syndrome.

Products

- Phenergan Elixir (5 mg per 5 mL)
- Phenergan Nightime tablets (25 mg)
  both *Sanofi-Aventis*

- Sominex tablets (20 mg)
  Thornton & Ross

- Ziz tablets (10 mg)
- Ziz Forte tablets (25 mg)
  both *Chatfield Laboratories*

Adverse effects, interactions and cautions

See chapter on Motion sickness.

Efficacy

Little research appears to have been conducted on the efficacy of sedating antihistamines as hypnotics. A study on rats[1] concluded that H_1-antagonists are effective in mild-to-moderate insomnia as sedative–hypnotic drugs, and that promethazine was more potent than diphenhydramine. A double-blind, placebo-controlled, cross-over study[2] found that diphenhydramine improved various sleep parameters, including sleep latency, to a significantly higher degree than did placebo. In addition, patients taking diphenhydramine reported feeling more rested the following morning. A trial on elderly patients[3] reported that promethazine was an effective hypnotic.

TREATMENT – HERBAL SLEEP AID PRODUCTS

A number of herbal products are licensed as General sale list medicines for the relief of restlessness and for promotion of relaxation and sleep. As is generally the case with herbal medicines, most are mixtures of several constituents. The constituents occurring most frequently are discussed below.

Herbal constituents

Hops

The compound 2-methyl-3-buten-2-ol extracted from hops (*Humulus lupulus*, Cannabinaceae), has been shown to possess narcotic properties in mice, and the plant is reported[4] to exhibit hypnotic and sedative actions in humans. Hops have been claimed to improve sleep disturbance when taken in association with valerian (see below). Hops are thought to be non-toxic in small doses, but their sedative action may potentiate the effects of other sedative therapy and alcohol.

Valerian

Valerian (*Valeriana officinalis*, Valerianaceae) contains valerenic acid, which has been shown to inhibit the enzyme system responsible for the metabolism of gamma-aminobutyric acid (GABA). Increased GABA is associated with a decrease in central nervous system (CNS) activity, and CNS depression has been observed in mice after injection of a valerian extract. A systematic review[5] indicated that valerian had some beneficial effects as a hypnotic, but evidence was sparse and limited. Valerian appears to be safe in use.

Passionflower

Passionflower *(Passiflora incarnata*, Passifloraceae) contains maltol and ethylmaltol, which have been shown to cause sedation and to increase the length of hexobarbital-induced sleeping time in laboratory mice. Passionflower also contains constituents that cause CNS stimulation, but the sedative effects appear to predominate. No adverse effects of the herb have been reported.

Jamaica dogwood

Studies with Jamaica dogwood (*Piscidia erythrina*, Leguminosae) in animals have shown weak cannabinoid and sedative properties, but no trials in humans appear to have been conducted. In *in vitro* and *in vivo* animal studies, Jamaica dogwood has been reported to strongly depress the activity of uterine muscle; use during pregnancy and lactation is therefore not recommended.

Wild lettuce

Wild lettuce (*Lactuca virosa*, Asteraceae/Compositae) has been reported to have mild sedative, analgesic and hypnotic properties, but this has not been scientifically demonstrated in humans.

Dosage

Recommended dosage varies from product to product, some being taken at bedtime, others in the early evening and at bedtime, and others three times daily.

Product examples

- Kalms Sleep tablets
  GR Lane

- Natrasleep tablets
  Chefaro UK

- Nodoff Passiflora tablets
- Nodoff mixture
  both *Potter's*

- Nytol Herbal tablets
  GSK Consumer Healthcare

- Slumber tablets
  Seven Seas

- Valerina Night-Time tablets
  Chemist Brokers Healthcare

A good night's sleep can often be achieved without resort to drugs, and pharmacists can offer practical advice to patients. Wherever possible, the underlying cause of insomnia, such as pain or anxiety, should be identified and addressed, and appropriate referrals made where necessary. Sleep aids should only be recommended to help re-establish a regular pattern of sleep and should be used for only a short period – 10 days at most.

The following advice can be given to aid sleep without the use of drugs.

- Wind down and relax towards the end of the evening. Do not do anything mentally stimulating within 90 minutes of bedtime. Gentle exercise, such as a short walk, just before bedtime, often helps.
- Do not sleep or doze during the evening. Do not go to bed until you feel tired and ready for sleep.
- Do not eat a large meal or have tea or coffee before bedtime. Do not drink alcohol; it may cause drowsiness but its effect is short-lived. A milky drink is often relaxing.
- Make sure that the bedroom and bed are warm and comfortable.
- Once in bed, put out the light immediately; do not read or watch television.
- Once the light is out, just relax, perhaps thinking of something pleasant and relaxing. Try to put any worries aside. Do not try to force yourself to sleep, let it come naturally.
- Aim to get up at the same time every day until a sleep pattern is restored.
- If you have not fallen asleep after 20 minutes, get up and do something relaxing and go back to bed when you feel sleepy. Do the same if you wake in the middle of the night and cannot get back to sleep.
- Remember that if you have naps during the day you will need to sleep less at night.
- Many people need much less than 8 hours' sleep per night.

PRODUCT SELECTION POINTS

- Non-drug strategies should be used for dealing with chronic insomnia where no specific cause can be identified.
- Diphenhydramine and promethazine appear to be effective in promoting sleep. 'Hangover' drowsiness the following morning may be a problem, particularly with promethazine.
- There is some evidence that herbal sleep aids are effective, but the same potential problem of psychological dependence exists for herbal products as for other hypnotics.
- Promethazine elixir is licensed for non-prescription use in children over 2 years of age, but should only be used as a last resort, when a cause has been clearly identified, and for a short period.
- Over-the-counter hypnotic products should only be recommended for occasional short periods and when a clear cause of stress can be identified. For sleeplessness due to any other reason, the cause should be identified and treated.

PRODUCT RECOMMENDATIONS

Temporary sleep disturbance associated with an identified change in sleeping pattern or short-term stress-related cause – diphenhydramine or a herbal sleep aid.

REFERENCES

1. Saitou K, Kaneko Y, Sugimoto Y, *et al.* Slow wave sleep-inducing effects of first generation H1-antagonists. *Biol Pharm Bull* 1999; 22: 1079–1082.
2. Rickels K, Morris RJ, Newman H, *et al.* Diphenhydramine in insomniac family practice patients: a double-blind study. *J Clin Pharmacol* 1983; 23: 234–342.
3. Viukari M, Miettinen P. Diazepam, promethazine and propiomazine as hypnotics in elderly inpatients. *Neuropsychobiology* 1984; 12: 134–137.
4. Muller-Limmroth W, Ehrenstein W. Experimental studies of the effects of Seda-Kneipp on the sleep of sleep disturbed subjects; implications for the treatment of different sleep disturbances. *Med Klin* 1977; 72: 1119–1125.
5. Stevinson C, Ernst E. Valerian for insomnia: a systematic review of randomized clinical trials. *Sleep Med* 2000; 1: 91–99.

Threadworm and roundworm

Threadworm (also known as pinworm) infection causes enterobiasis, the only commonly occurring helminth infection in the UK. Roundworm infections have a much lower incidence, and are likely to have been contracted abroad rather than in the UK.

Threadworm

Threadworm (*Enterobius vermicularis*) infection is estimated to affect up to 40% of children by the time they are 10 years old and is also contracted by adults, but the incidence is lower. The condition can often be diagnosed by the pharmacist and suitable non-prescription treatment recommended.

Threadworms are initially acquired through swallowing eggs, which hatch and mature in the small intestine. After copulating, the males die and the females migrate to the caecum and anus at night to lay their eggs in the perianal area, attaching them to the skin with a sticky, highly irritant fluid. Some eggs hatch there and the emergent worms return to the rectum to mature. The intense itching caused by the sticky secretion provokes scratching by the host, and eggs are transferred on to the fingers. Infection is passed on or perpetuated through picking up eggs on the fingers, followed by ingestion. Infection is transmitted either by direct contact between individuals or from contaminated surfaces or objects, as eggs can remain viable for several weeks outside the human host under suitable conditions.

Infection is recognised by sighting the whitish worms, which are about 10 mm in length, on the stools after defecation and sometimes around the anus, and also from the intense perianal itching that they cause. Enterobiasis is treated with mebendazole or piperazine, both of which are available without prescription.

Roundworm

Roundworm infection (ascariasis) has a much lower incidence, and is likely to have been contracted abroad rather than in the UK. The consequences of infection are potentially much more serious than with enterobiasis and, if suspected, the patient should be referred to a doctor. The condition is included here because the same products are used to treat threadworms and roundworms, and, as they cost less than a prescription charge, patients may be recommended by their doctor to buy piperazine over the counter as treatment for roundworm infection.

Roundworm infection is much less easy to identify than threadworm infection, and is potentially serious. Eggs of the common roundworm (*Ascaris lumbricoides*) are ingested in food or water contaminated with faeces, and hatch in the intestine. The larvae pass into the blood stream and lymphatic system and migrate via the lung, liver, trachea and oesophagus back to the intestine. Light infestations are usually symptomless, but heavy infestations produce serious gastrointestinal symptoms and are sometimes fatal. Ascariasis is rare in the UK and specialised medical expertise may be necessary to diagnose it.

Piperazine is licensed for non-prescription sale for the treatment of roundworm infections, but mebendazole may only be used for this infection on prescription.

TREATMENT

Mebendazole

Mode of action

Mebendazole is a benzimidazole derivative which disrupts parasite energy metabolism by causing selective destruction of cytoplasmic microtubules in tegumental and intestinal cells; it irreversibly inhibits glucose uptake and causes immobilisation and death of the parasite within 3 days of administration. It also binds to tubulin, a protein required by the parasite for the uptake of nutrients.

Mebendazole is effective against both threadworms and round-worms, but for non-prescription use is licensed only for the former. It is poorly absorbed from the human gastrointestinal tract, and the small proportion of a dose that is absorbed is almost entirely elimi-nated from the body following first-pass metabolism in the liver. Mebendazole has been in use for 30 years and is an established treat-ment throughout the world. Clinical trials have shown it to be highly effective.[1-4]

Dosage

The dose for adults and children over 2 years of age is a single 100 mg dose. Treatment failures are rare, but re-infection is possible, in which case a second dose should be given after 2–3 weeks. Mebendazole is not recommended for children under 2 years of age.

Adverse effects and cautions

Side-effects are unlikely at the dose used for threadworm infection; transient diarrhoea and abdominal pain have been rarely reported in patients with heavy infections. Hypersensitivity reactions also occur rarely.

Mebendazole has shown embryotoxic and teratogenic activity in rats, but not in other species. When it has been used in pregnant women, even during the first trimester, the incidence of malformations or spontaneous abortion has been no higher than in the general popu-lation.[5,6] However, the drug is not licensed for use in pregnancy or breastfeeding when sold without prescription.

Interactions

Cimetidine inhibits the metabolism of mebendazole in the liver, increasing blood plasma concentrations. Phenytoin and carba-mazepine induce enzyme metabolism and have been found to reduce serum mebendazole levels. However, since mebendazole exerts its effect directly within the gut, and the drug is poorly absorbed, these interactions are unlikely to have any clinical significance.

Products

- Ovex tablets and suspension
  McNeil

- Pripsen mebendazole tablets
  Thornton & Ross

Piperazine

Mode of action

Piperazine has been in use as an enterobiacide for about 50 years and, until 1989, when mebendazole was reclassified from Prescription-only medicine to Pharmacy medicine, piperazine was the only anthelmintic available without prescription. However, mebendazole is now usually the first-choice treatment.[7] Piperazine is active against both threadworms and roundworms, and can be sold without prescription for infections caused by either.

Piperazine acts by blocking the response of worm muscle to acetylcholine, and by interfering with the permeability of cell membranes to ions that regulate the cell membrane resting potential. Flaccid paralysis results, and the paralysed worms are then expelled from the gut by peristalsis. Piperazine is readily absorbed from the gastrointestinal tract, but is almost completely metabolised and excreted through the kidney within 24 hours.

Dosage

Several salts of piperazine are used as anthelmintics, but only the phosphate is available in the UK.

Piperazine phosphate is presented as a powder in sachets containing 4 g, together with standardised senna, which acts as a laxative to facilitate the expulsion of the paralysed worms.

Doses for threadworms are as follows: adults and children over 6 years of age, one sachet; children up to 6 years of age – one level

5 mL spoonful of sachet contents; infants aged 3–12 months (treatment only on medical advice) – one level 2.5 mL spoonful of sachet contents.

The powder should be stirred into a small glass of water or milk and drunk immediately. Because the life cycle of the threadworm is about 30 days and some worms may be in the larval stage when the first dose is taken, the manufacturer recommends that a second dose be taken after 14 days to eliminate the possibility of re-infection.

For roundworms, the initial dose is the same as for threadworms; follow-up doses every month for 3 months may be advised to prevent re-infection.

Adverse effects and cautions

Adverse effects are rare at dosages within normal therapeutic ranges. Allergic-type symptoms have been reported and mild gastrointestinal disturbances in sensitive individuals. Neurotoxic reactions resulting in convulsions have occasionally occurred in patients with neurological or renal abnormalities, and piperazine should not be used in patients with severe renal or hepatic dysfunction or a history of epilepsy.

The drug is not contraindicated in pregnancy, but isolated instances of congenital malformations in babies whose mothers had taken piperazine while pregnant have been reported, although no causal relationship has been established. Manufacturers therefore advise that piperazine should be taken in pregnancy only if strictly necessary and under medical supervision, and should be avoided altogether in the first trimester. The drug is excreted in breast milk, although no untoward effects in infants have been reported. However, it is recommended that mothers taking piperazine should not breast-feed for at least 8 hours following a dose.

Interactions

Caution is advised in administering piperazine to patients taking phenothiazines or tricyclic antidepressants; this is based on a single reported case of an interaction causing convulsions, and also on studies in animals.

Product

- Pripsen piperazine phosphate powder (with senna)
  Thornton & Ross

PRACTICAL ADVICE

In addition to use of an anthelmintic, whether mebendazole or piperazine, pharmacists should advise patients to take the following measures to prevent re-infection and transmission of threadworms.

- When infection is detected in any member of a family, the whole family should be treated with an anthelmintic, as other members may be in the early stages of infection, although asymptomatic.
- As infection is easily passed on through contact, scrupulous hygiene should be observed. All members of the family should wash their hands thoroughly before preparing, handling or eating food. As eggs can be harboured under the finger nails, they should be kept short and scrubbed with a nailbrush when the hands are washed.
- Children with threadworms should wear underpants under pyjamas at night to prevent them transferring eggs to their fingers if they scratch during sleep.
- Infected individuals should have a bath or shower on getting up each morning, to wash away any eggs laid overnight.

PRODUCT SELECTION POINTS

- Mebendazole is the treatment of choice for threadworms. It is suitable for all patients over 2 years old, with the same single dose for all ages. It is almost completely free from adverse effects and, apart from pregnancy, there are no contraindications.

- Mebendazole is not licensed for non-prescription use in children under 2 years of age, but piperazine can be used from the age of 1 year. Children under 1 year of age should be treated under medical supervision.
- Neither mebendazole nor piperazine can be supplied without prescription to pregnant women.
- Piperazine, but not mebendazole, is available without prescription for the treatment of roundworms, but it should only be supplied following medical diagnosis.
- Stringent hygiene precautions should be taken to prevent re-infection and transmission of threadworms.

PRODUCT RECOMMENDATIONS

- For threadworms, the first choice for adults and children over 2 years – mebendazole.
- For children aged 1–2 years – piperazine phosphate sachets.
- Piperazine may be sold without prescription for roundworm infections, but supply should only be made following medical diagnosis.

REFERENCES

1. St Georgiev V. Chemotherapy of enterobiasis (oxyuriasis). *Expert Opin Pharmacother* 2001; 2: 267–275.
2. Seo BS, Cho SY, Kang SY, Chai JY. Anthelmintic efficacy of methyl-5-benzoylbenzimidazole-2-carbamate (mebendazole) against multiple helminthic infections. *Kisaengchunghak Chapchi* 1977; 15: 11–16.
3. Cho SY, Ahn YR, Ryang YS, Seo BS. Evaluation of anthelmintic treatment of *Enterobius vermicularis* infection in highly endemic population by prolonged observation. *Kisaengchunghak Chapchi* 1977; 15: 100–108.
4. Lormans JA, Wesel AJ, Vanparus OF. Mebendazole (R 17635) in enterobiasis. A clinical trial in mental retardates. *Chemotherapy* 1975; 21: 255–260.
5. Diav-Citrin O, Shechtman S, Arnon J, *et al*. Pregnancy outcome after gestational exposure to mebendazole: a prospective controlled cohort study. *Am J Obstet Gynecol* 2003; 188: 282–285.

6. Acs N, Banhidy F, Puho E, Czeizel AE. Population-based case-control study of mebendazole in pregnant women for birth outcomes. *Congenit Anom* 2005; 45: 85–88.
7. Sweetman SC, ed. *Martindale: The complete drug reference,* 34th edn. London: Pharmaceutical Press, 2005; 112.

Vaginal candidiasis

Vaginal candidiasis (thrush) is the most common vaginal infection, with about half of all women between 16 and 60 years of age experiencing an infection at some time, and more than one-third having at least one infection each year. It can be successfully treated with azole preparations, which are available without prescription. Products based on iodine are also available, but they are less effective and less convenient to use.

CAUSE

Vaginal candidiasis is caused by a yeast, *Candida albicans*, usually a harmless inhabitant of the gastrointestinal tract, skin and vagina, which overgrows opportunistically to cause infections when conditions allow.

All vaginal infections other than candidiasis require treatment under medical supervision.

TREATMENT – AZOLES

Compounds available

Compounds available are:

- Imidazoles
    - clotrimazole
    - econazole

- Triazole
    - fluconazole

Mode of action

Azoles are synthetic antimycotic agents, which act by inhibiting replication of the yeast cells through interfering with the synthesis of ergosterol, the main sterol in the yeast cell membrane. As a further consequence, the transformation of candidal yeast cells into hyphae, the invasive and pathogenic form of the organism, is also inhibited. Preparations of clotrimazole and econazole are applied locally; fluconazole is taken orally.

Imidazoles for local application are weak bases and have to remain in the non-ionised form in order to be active; they therefore work best in an alkaline medium and should not be used in the presence of acidifying agents. The use of live yoghurt is sometimes advocated as a 'natural' treatment for vaginal candidiasis. This advice has a rational basis, as Lactobacilli in the yoghurt convert glycogen present in the vagina into lactic acid, which reduces the adherence of the yeast cells to the walls of the vagina and inhibits their growth. However, by creating an acid medium, the use of yoghurt would reduce the effectiveness of imidazoles, so the two should not be administered together. Yoghurt may sometimes be helpful for vaginal candidiasis, but it is much less effective than treatment with imidazoles and is messier to use. A systematic review[1] found no evidence of effectiveness, but that oral yoghurt may cause gastrointestinal disturbance in people with lactose intolerance.

A large body of evidence, brought together in *Clinical Evidence*[2] and a Cochrane Review,[3] shows that azole antifungals, particularly those licensed for non-prescription use in the UK, are effective and safe treatments for vulvovaginal candidiasis, with clinical and mycological cure rates of 80–95%. The Cochrane Review concluded that there was no difference in relative effectiveness between oral and intravaginal antifungals and little difference in safety profile. It considered oral administration to be the preferred route, although the greater convenience of oral preparations needed to be balanced against their higher cost.

Topical preparations are formulated as creams, pessaries and vaginal tablets and courses of treatment range from a single dose to six applications. Creams are also available for application to the vulva to treat irritation. In addition, some medical authorities consider that application of such a cream to the partner's penis is useful in preventing re-infection, although there is no consensus on this, and little or no evidence of the effectiveness of treating asymptomatic male partners.[4] Systemic absorption of locally applied imidazoles is slight, with wide intersubject variation and there is no evidence of problems occurring from absorption during the short courses used for non-prescription treatment. Trials have indicated that single-dose formulations are as effective as longer courses, and they are preferred by patients on grounds of convenience.

Fluconazole is presented as a single-dose oral capsule. It is well absorbed when taken by mouth, reaching peak serum concentrations within 1–2 hours of administration; the elimination half-life is about 30 hours.

Administration and dosage

Night-time use is recommended for intravaginal preparations, as the patient will be lying down for several hours, thus allowing the drug a chance to act and avoiding the problems of seepage and loss that would occur if the patient were upright and moving around. Oral fluconazole is more convenient from this point of view and can be taken at any time of day.

- Clotrimazole
  - vaginal cream (10%): 5 g at night as a single dose
  - pessaries: 1 × 500 mg as a single dose at night; 1 × 100 mg nightly for 6 nights or 1 × 200 mg nightly for 3 nights
  - topical cream (1% and 2%): apply to the anogenital area two or three times a day.

There appears to be no published evidence that 2% cream is more effective than 1% in treating external symptoms.

- Econazole – topical cream (1%): apply to the anogenital area twice daily
- Fluconazole – oral capsule (150 mg): one single dose.

Adverse effects, cautions and contraindications

Burning and irritation may occur with the topical imidazoles, and contact dermatitis has been reported. However, it is thought that the amount of drug absorbed during the short courses used to treat vaginal candidiasis is insufficient to cause adverse systemic effects. The bases used in some preparations damage latex condoms and diaphragms; package inserts provide relevant information.

Adverse effects associated with oral fluconazole are mainly gastrointestinal, including abdominal pain, diarrhoea, nausea and vomiting and flatulence. Teratogenicity has occurred with high doses of fluconazole in animals, and the drug is also excreted in breast milk. The licensing conditions for all non-prescription azoles prohibit their use in pregnant and breastfeeding women. Fluconazole should also be used with caution in patients with impaired renal or hepatic function.

In order to minimise any risk of adverse effects or inappropriate use, the Medicines and Healthcare Products Regulatory Agency (MHRA) has imposed a number of conditions and prohibitions on the supply of azoles without prescription.

- They should only be supplied to women who have had vaginal candidiasis diagnosed previously by a doctor. This is to exclude the possibility that a patient may be suffering from another type of vaginal infection that would have to be treated with drugs available only on prescription. If a woman has had a previous diagnosis of candidiasis, she should recognise the symptoms.
- They should not be supplied to women who have had more than two attacks of candidiasis in the previous 6 months, as this could indicate an underlying cause, such as diabetes, which needs to be investigated.
- They should not be supplied to women under 16 or over 60 years of age. Vaginal candidiasis is rare in these age groups,

as the oestrogen necessary to create the conditions that favour the growth of *C. albicans* is lacking. However, lack of oestrogen increases susceptibility to other vaginal infections.

- They should not be supplied to pregnant or breastfeeding women. Teratogenicity has occurred with high doses of fluconazole and other systemic imidazoles in animals, and although there is no evidence of such an effect with locally administered preparations or a single oral dose, the MHRA has decided that the potential risks should be considered by a patient's doctor before a supply is made.

- They should not be supplied to patients reporting symptoms such as vaginal bleeding, dysuria, pain in the lower abdomen or sores or blisters in the genital area, which might indicate conditions that are more serious than candidiasis.

- They should not be supplied to patients with a previous history of sexually transmitted disease or who have been in contact with a partner with such a history, as other infections apart from candidiasis may be present.

Interactions

Fluconazole interacts with a number of drugs, including those metabolised by cytochrome P450 isoenzyme CYP3A4. It can increase plasma concentrations of several drugs that have narrow therapeutic margins, including warfarin, theophylline and phenytoin. It also increases plasma concentrations of sulphonylureas, tacrolimus and ciclosporin. Rifampicin increases the metabolism of fluconazole, resulting in reduced plasma concentrations. However, these interactions are unlikely to be clinically significant with a single dose of fluconazole.

Products

- Clotrimazole
  - — Canesten cream (topical: 1%)
  - — Canesten Thrush Cream (topical: 2%)
  - — Canesten Cream Combi (vaginal cream: 10%, topical: 2%)
  - — Canesten Internal Cream (vaginal cream: 10%)
  - — Canesten pessaries (100 mg, 200 mg, 500 mg)
  - — Canesten Combi pessary & cream (500 mg pessary and topical cream 2%)

    all *Bayer*

- Econazole
  - — Ecostatin Cream (topical: 1%)

    Bristol-Myers Squibb
  - — Pevaryl cream (topical: 1%)

    Janssen-Cilag

- Fluconazole
  - — Canesten oral capsule (150 mg)
  - — Canesten Oral & Cream Duo (150 mg capsule, topical: 2% cream)

    Bayer
  - — Diflucan One oral capsule (150 mg)

    Pfizer Consumer Healthcare

Mode of action

Povidone-iodine is an iodophore in which povidone, a vinyl polymer, acts as a carrier for iodine, allowing its gradual release for anti-microbial and antiseptic effect. It is less potent than preparations containing free iodine but is also less toxic. It has activity against a wide range of microorganisms, including fungi, but is less effective than the azoles and requires twice-daily administration for up to 14 days. It should not be used in pregnancy or during breastfeeding, because of the risk of iodine interfering with infant thyroid function. There is some evidence from clinical trials[5,6] to show that povidone-iodine pessaries are safe and reasonably effective.

Products and dosage

- Betadine vaginal pessaries: 200 mg – one inserted twice daily
- Betadine VC vaginal cleansing kit: 10% solution with a special bottle and vaginal applicator – for daily use diluted as a douche
- Betadine vaginal gel (10%): 5 g daily in association with pessaries or douche
  all *Medlock*

PRODUCT SELECTION POINTS

- All imidazole compounds for local application appear to be equally effective.
- Single-dose topical formulations are as effective as longer courses and obviate compliance problems.
- Single-dose oral fluconazole is as effective as preparations for local use and is generally preferred by patients. Possible disadvantages are the higher price and the slightly higher risk of adverse effects resulting from greater systemic absorption.

PRODUCT RECOMMENDATIONS

- A single-dose imidazole pessary, vaginal tablet or vaginal cream, or fluconazole oral capsule (best avoided in patients taking medication with which it interacts).
- A topical cream for use on the external genitalia, if necessary.

REFERENCES

1. Van Kessel K, Assefi N, Marrazzo J, Eckert L. Common complementary and alternative therapies for yeast vaginitis and bacterial vaginosis: a systematic review. *Obstet Gynecol Surv* 2003; 58: 351–358.

2. *Clinical Evidence*. BMJ Publishing. (www.clinicalevidence.com/) accessed February 2006.

3. Watson MC, Grimshaw JM, Bond CM, *et al.* Oral versus intra-vaginal imidazole and triazole anti-fungal treatment of uncomplicated vulvovaginal candidiasis (thrush). *The Cochrane Library,* issue 3. Chichester, UK: John Wiley & Sons, 2001 (www.thecochranelibrary.com).

4. Fong IW. The value of treating the sexual partners of women with recurrent vaginal candidiasis with ketoconazole. *Genitourin Med* 1992; 68: 174–176.

5. Petersen EE, Weissenbacher ER, Hengst P, *et al.* Local treatment of vaginal infections of varying etiology with dequalinium chloride or povidone iodine. A randomised, double-blind, active-controlled, multicentric clinical study. *Arzneimittelforschung* 2002; 52: 706–715.

6. Yu H, Tak-Yin M. The efficacy of povidone-iodine pessaries in a short, low-dose treatment regime on candidal, trichomonal and non-specific vaginitis. *Postgrad Med J* 1993; 69 (Suppl 3): S58–S61.

Vaginitis and vaginal dryness

Vaginitis and vaginal dryness are the result of atrophic changes that reduce secretions and alter their pH, increasing susceptibility to infection. Sexual intercourse can become painful.

Vaginitis and vaginal dryness can be caused by oestrogen deficiency following the menopause.

For many women, vaginitis and vaginal dryness are avoided or remedied by use of hormone replacement therapy or intravaginal oestrogen preparations, which are available on prescription. However, hormonal therapy is unsuitable for some women, and others choose not to use it. Non-prescription products are available to counteract problems of vaginal dryness and reduction in acidity.

Products, actions and use

Products available are inert aqueous gels.

K-Y Jelly (J&J MSD) provides short-acting lubrication and can be applied immediately before sexual intercourse.

Replens MD (Anglian) is a bioadhesive product containing polycarbophil, a polymer that holds up to 60 times its weight in water, and has the ability to adhere to vaginal epithelial cells. The manufacturer claims that an application stays in place for up to 72 hours until the cells to which it adheres are naturally discarded, and that as well as lubricating, the product moisturises the vaginal walls by driving water into the underlying cells. Polycarbophil is acidic and reduces vaginal pH to premenopausal levels, thereby increasing resistance to infection. Replens can be used three times a week continuously. Results of clinical trials[1,2] have shown that Replens is generally equivalent in safety and efficacy to vaginal oestrogen cream for post-menopausal vaginal dryness.

REFERENCES

1. Nachtigall LE. Comparative study: Replens versus local estrogen in menopausal women. *Fertil Steri.* 1994; 61: 178–180.
2. Bygdeman M, Swahn ML. Replens versus dienoestrol cream in the symptomatic treatment of vaginal atrophy in postmenopausal women. *Maturitas* 1996; 23: 259–263.

Verrucas

(continued . . .)

Verrucas (plantar warts) are benign viral infections of the epidermis on the sole of the foot.

Verrucas are caused by the human papillomavirus and result in hyper-keratinisation. A verruca is simply a wart that has been compressed by the weight put upon it, and is painful because of pressure exerted on the nerve endings. Verrucas are most common in children, and although they resolve spontaneously, they are usually treated actively as resolution can take months or even years.

Treatment is by gradual removal of the hyperkeratotic skin layers and the viral core by keratolytic agents.

Several products are marketed for the removal of corns and calluses and also for warts and verrucas. Compounds used include:

- salicylic acid
- lactic acid
- podophyllum resin
- formaldehyde
- glutaraldehyde
- silver nitrate.

Salicylic acid

Mode of action

When used in the treatment of warts and verrucas, salicylic acid reduces viral numbers by mechanical removal of infected tissue. It also stimulates production of protective antibodies in response to the mildly irritant effect of the acid. Salicylic acid is a constituent of many wart and verruca treatments, alone and in combination with other ingredients. Some products are the same as those marketed for corns and calluses. A Cochrane review[1] concluded that simple topical treatments containing salicylic acid have a therapeutic effect in the treatment of warts, increasing complete wart clearance, successful treatment or loss of one or more warts after 6–12 weeks compared with placebo. In a comparative trial,[2] salicylic acid was found to have a high cure rate (84%) for simple plantar warts and to be as effective as cryotherapy for hand warts; a podophyllum treatment also had a high cure rate of 81%.

Product examples

- Salicylic Acid Collodion BP (12%: see chapter on Corns and Calluses)

- Bazuka Extra Strength (26% in a film-forming gel)
  Dendron

- Occlusal (26% in a polyacrylic vehicle)
  Alliance

- Scholl Verruca Removal System (medicated discs containing 40%)
- Scholl Seal and Heal Verruca Removal Gel (12.5% in a film-forming gel)
  both *SSL International*

- Verrugon (ointment containing 50%)
  Ransom

Lactic acid

Mode of action

Lactic acid has corrosive properties and is included with salicylic acid in several verruca products. It is claimed to enhance the effects of salicylic acid. Care must be taken that preparations do not spread onto unaffected skin.

Product examples

- Containing 16.7% lactic acid, with 16.7% salicylic acid in a collodion base
  — Duofilm
    Stiefel
  — Salactol wart paint
    Dermal

- Containing 4% lactic acid, with 11–12% salicylic acid in a film-forming gel
  — Bazuka
    Dendron
  — Cuplex gel
    Crawford
  — Salatac gel
    Dermal

Podophyllum resin

Mode of action and adverse effects

Podophyllum resin (podophyllin) is obtained from the dried rhizome of the May-apple (*Podophyllum peltatum*). It has a potent corrosive action, and for non-prescription use it is solely indicated for plantar warts. It is cytotoxic and a caustic and powerful skin irritant; care must be taken to confine its application to the verruca only. There have also been reports of teratogenicity and it is contraindicated in pregnancy.

Product

- Posalfilin ointment (20% podophyllum resin, plus 25% salicylic acid)
  Norgine

Formaldehyde

Mode of action

Formaldehyde has antiviral activity; it also has a direct anhidrotic action, drying the verruca and surrounding skin.

Products

- Veracur gel (0.75% formaldehyde in an aqueous gel base – a disadvantage is that it must be used twice daily)
  Typharm

- Solution of formaldehyde (3% – can be used for daily foot soaks if there are a large number of verrucas, although care must be taken to protect unaffected skin)

Glutaraldehyde

Mode of action

Glutaraldehyde has similar properties to formaldehyde. However, it appears to have no advantage over formaldehyde and may be a more potent skin sensitiser. It stains skin brown, but this fades once treatment is discontinued.

Product

- Glutarol Wart Paint (10%)
  Dermal

Silver nitrate

Mode of action

Silver nitrate is a caustic agent; it is used in the form of a stick or pencil (95% toughened with 5% potassium nitrate) to destroy warts, verrucas and other skin growths. Unlike other treatments for verrucas, silver nitrate pencil is used for only a short period; the manufacturer of the only commercially available product claims that three daily applications are sufficient, but that a maximum of six may be made. In a clinical trial,[3] silver nitrate stick completely or partially cured common warts in 69% of subjects, compared with 25% with placebo.

Product

There is only one product:

- Avoca Wart and Verruca Set
  Bray

Application and use

Removal of verrucas is achieved by a process of gradual abrading of the infected tissue, and the same basic method is used for all preparations. The following points of advice should be given to patients.

- Before application, gently rub away the top layer of skin with a file, emery board or pumice stone.

- Apply the preparation directly to the top of the verruca, taking precautions to confine it to that area.
- Cover the verruca with a plaster to encourage maceration and improve penetration of the medicament.
- Remove the plaster after 24 hours and file away the dead tissue on top of the verruca.
- Repeat the process daily until all trace of the verruca has been removed; this may take up to 3 months (except for silver nitrate – see above) but the verruca may regrow if all infected tissue has not been removed.

PRODUCT SELECTION POINTS

- Salicylic acid has been shown to be an effective treatment for plantar and hand warts, and collodion-based products provide a convenient and efficient method of application.
- There is little published evidence of effectiveness for other agents used in the treatment of verrucas and warts.

PRODUCT RECOMMENDATIONS

Salicylic Acid Collodion BP or similar preparation.

REFERENCES

1. Gibbs S, Harvey I, Sterling J, *et al*. Local treatments for cutaneous warts: systematic review. *The Cochrane Library*, issue 3. Chichester, UK: John Wiley & Sons, 2004 (www.thecochranelibrary.com).
2. Bunney MH, Nolan MW, Williams DA An assessment of methods of treating viral warts by comparative treatment trials based on a standard design. *Br J Dermatol* 1976; 94: 667–679.
3. Yazar S, Basaran E. Efficacy of silver nitrate pencils in the treatment of common warts. *J Dermatol* 1994; 21: 329–333.

Warts

Warts are benign growths caused by viral infection. They occur most frequently on the hands and fingers, and less commonly on the elbows and knees. Cutaneous, or common warts as they are more usually known, can occur at any age but incidence peaks at 12–16 years and declines after 20 years of age. They mostly occur in children and young adults, with an overall incidence of 10%. A study of school children[1] found that 4% of 11-year-old children had warts, but 93% of these no longer had warts by the age of 16 years.

CAUSE

Like verrucas, warts are caused by the human papillomavirus and, apart from their location and the fact that they are usually painless because they are not compressed, they are identical to verrucas (see chapter on Verrucas).

TREATMENT

Treatment is essentially the same as for verrucas (see chapter on Verrucas) and nearly all the products available are licensed for both warts and verrucas.

Of the products listed under verrucas, most are licensed for treatment of both common and plantar warts. Some are licensed exclusively for the latter because they are presented as kits containing plasters or pads to relieve pain resulting from pressure exerted by body weight on plantar warts. Only Posalfilin (Norgine) is restricted to treatment of plantar warts by virtue of one its constituents – podophyllum resin.

REFERENCE

1. Williams HC, Pottier A, Strachan D. The descriptive epidemiology of warts in British schoolchildren. *Br J Dermatol* 1993; 128: 504–511.

Index

Proprietary drug names are in *italics*.